FOOD SCIENCE AND TECHNOLOGY

SEED OIL

PRODUCTION, USES AND BENEFITS

FOOD SCIENCE AND TECHNOLOGY

Additional books in this series can be found on Nova's website under the Series tab.

Additional e-books in this series can be found on Nova's website under the e-BookS tab.

FOOD SCIENCE AND TECHNOLOGY

SEED OIL

PRODUCTION, USES AND BENEFITS

NGUYEN KHANH DIEU HONG
EDITOR

nova
science publishers
New York

Additional color graphics may be available in the e-book version of this book.

Library of Congress Cataloging-in-Publication Data
Names: Hong Nguyen Khanh, Dieu, editor.
Title: Seed oil : production, uses and benefits / editor, Hong Nguyen Khanh
Dieu (Department of Petrochemical-Technology, School of Chemical Engineering, Hanoi University of Science and Technology, Hanoi, Vietnam).
Description: Hauppauge, New York : Nova Science Publisher's, Inc., 2018. | Series: Food science and technology | Includes index.
Identifiers: LCCN 2018013605 (print) | LCCN 2018014949 (ebook) | ISBN
9781536135619 (ebook) | ISBN 9781536135602 (hardcover) | ISBN 9781536135619 (ebook)
Subjects: LCSH: Vegetable oils in human nutrition.
Classification: LCC QP144.O44 (ebook) | LCC QP144.O44 S45 2018 (print) | DDC 613.2/84--dc23
LC record available at https://lccn.loc.gov/2018013605

Published by Nova Science Publishers, Inc. † New York

CONTENTS

PREFACE

Vegetable oils have been regarded as a new generation feedstock that requires strengthening and developing in the near future. In this book, various kinds of seed oil derived feedstock including, moringa oleifera seed oil, neem seed oil, calophyllum inophyllum seed oil, grape seed oil, argan oil and rubber seed oil are introduced in terms of their production, applications and development in a variety of sectors such as industries, healthcare, cosmetics, medicine or functional food, bio-pesticide and biofuels. These uses all bring considerable benefits to the economy, social development and environmental protection. The book content reviews different aspects of refining and applying processes for each seed oil, as well as reveals a number of research results published by the authors of each chapter. Upon further consideration, all these seed oils are categorized as the second generation feedstock; they do not compete with food security and have higher productivity compared to the others. Therefore, they could play a crucial role in making new products like biofuels, green fuels and so on, enhancing the performance of the old products and processes such as synthetic pesticide production, hydraulic or lubricant application. Thus, they either partially or completely replace the improper feedstock, including fossil sources, first generation vegetable oils and fats, to name but a few.

Chapter 1 - During the last few decades, *Moringa oleifera* seeds have gained enormous scientific attention. Indeed, the rapid growth of this tree, even under hard climatic conditions, its low demand for soil nutrients and watering, associated with its high production of seeds (more than one harvest a year) with a high oil yield (up to 44%), makes its production and development easy and reliable for the industry as a new source of oil for edible and non-edible purposes. In the past, *Moringa oleifera* seed oil was used mostly in the dermocosmetic field, including in perfumes, skin lotions and ointments to treat disorders and damages imposed by the extremes of desert weather conditions. Scientifics evidences of its good quality and suitability for edible purposes came latter, with a particular interest on its high mono-unsaturated to saturated fatty acids ratio, included in the category of natural high oleic oils, as olive oil, and therefore desirable in terms of nutrition, health and even technological applications. It is also rich in micronutrients such as tocopherols and phytosterols, which have demonstrated strong *in vivo* antioxidant activity, and are beneficial in the prevention and treatment of several medical disorders and ailments

In this regards, a review regrouping the most pertinent information on Moringa tree propagation, as well as the composition, production, uses and health benefits of its seed oil, would be of a great interests and advantageous for further investigations and curious readers.

Chapter 2 - The Agrochemicals have been conventional in the control of Agricultural pests. These are Synthetic pesticides used during crop production to control pests. They are very useful in crop production, however it has been noticed that the use of this form of pesticide has effects which are detrimental to man and his environment. On man, there are its recorded effects on the immune system, the endocrine gland as well as the reproductive tract. Some of which includes respiratory organ's malfunction, memory disorder, birth defects, miscarriages, cancer etc. Recorded effects on the environment include land, water and air pollution. In view of these problems, the exploration of ecologically safe pest control alternatives in crop production becomes imperative. Consequently, there has been an increased research attention on the use of natural compounds as a poisoning option to replace agro-chemicals. These natural compounds also known as botanical insecticides which the Neem seed oil is one of them constitute desirable alternatives to the synthetic pesticides. They are best suited for use in organic food production in industrialized countries. Nevertheless, they can still play a much greater role in the developing countries as a new class of eco-friendly products for pest control. These botanical pesticides should be incorporated in the pest management programs. When, this is done, they can serve as alternatives to synthetic pesticides, or used in combination them, or more so in rotation with other pesticides. The application of the above options could delay the development of control resistance in pests. The plant based insecticides induce acute toxicity to pests which deters them from causing great economic losses at the pre- and post- harvest stages of crop production. The Neem amongst other plant species is the most researched and commercially exploited in pest management. The substances with pesticidal properties are found in all parts of the Neem tree, however, the greatest concentration of it is found in the seed. The Neem seed contains an active ingredient called the Azadirachtin which consists of more than 25 different but closely related compounds. It is extracted from the seed kernel in the form of oil, cake or powder. This Neem Seed Kernel Extracts (NSKE) viz-a-viz the Neem Seed Oil (NO) and the Neem Cake (NC) are used in various fields and horticultural crops for pest management. The Azadirachtin was reported to be active against over 550 insect species. The NO is a powerful and natural insecticide capable of disrupting the life cycle of insects at all stages. Its efficacy and availability makes it a great resource for the poor farmers. The modes of action of NSKE on insect pests include direct effect on insect reproduction which is manifested in their growth reduction, increased mortality rate, abnormal and delayed moults. This research explains the production, uses and benefits of the Neem seed oil.

Chapter 3 - *Calophyllum inophyllum* is a mangrove plant species from the family of *Calophyllaceae*. It is a native of southern coastal India to Malesia, northern Australia, East Africa, and the Pacific Islands. It produces fruits at age of 7-58 years. Fruit and seed productions are 60-220 and 50-150 kg/tree/year, respectively. Most researchers were focused on conversion of *C. inophyllum* oil into biodiesel due to its high oil content. Therefore, the aim of this chapter is to discuss the production, refining, and utilization of *C. inophyllum* seed oil as well as its future perspective. Oil content (%) and yield (kg oil per ha) of several edible and non-edible oils were presented. The development of new refining techniques of *C. inophyllum* seed oil has gained increasing importance in the biodiesel and pharmaceutical industries, due to its content of economically-valuable compounds, the necessity of environmental friendly process, and energy security. There are several different methodologies of separation and purification for improving the quality of *C. inophyllum* oil purity (triacylglycerol), such as chemical, physical and batchwise solvent-solvent extraction. Moreover, fatty acids in triacylglycerol (TAG) are the key factor for the quality of oil due to the *cis* and *trans* configuration. It is of great interest if new utilization of *C. inophyllum* seed oil is available. This oil may have a potential to be used as an edible oil after treatments. However, further clinical studies are needed.

Chapter 4 - During wine production, formation of biomass residue (peel, seed and grape stems) occurs and thus constitute a problem from an environmental point of view. Nevertheless, this residue may be reused with the purpose of obtaining products with beneficial properties for Human beings as well as for the environment. Seeds from grapes can be used in the food industry to obtain oils. This use makes of them a value-added food due to its richness in linoleic acid, vitamin E, and phytosterols responsible for several biological properties such as antioxidant, anti-inflammatory, and anti-hypercholesterolemia activities. In the chapter, the main procedures to obtain grape seed oils, their chemical composition and biological properties will be reviewed.

Chapter 5 - The Argan tree (*Arganiaspinosa* (L.) Skeels; Sapotaceae) is a slow-growing tree exclusively endemic to the barren lands of southwest Morocco. The oil extracted from argan seed is almost exclusively produced in southwestern Morocco. It is reputed for its unique savor and its several pharmacological and cosmetic properties.

The oil extraction requires a tedious multistep process. The first step is a careful fruit drying. This oil extraction requires a prolonged hand-malaxing of an aqueous argan kernel dow. The extraction yield can reach 35% and more. The extraction has been improved by the use of electric screw-presses, which allows the discontinuation of the hand-malaxing step, resulting in as much as 60-percent extraction yield.

Virgin edible argan oil is a main component of the Amazigh diet. It is prepared from slightly and carefully roasted kernels and it is copper-colored with a slight hazelnut taste. Health benefits of argan oil are attributed to its composition of unsaponiable fraction mainly rich in tocopherols. Argan oil has hepatoprotective, antiproliferative anti-diabetic properties and also cancer preventive potential. It is used in beauty and cosmetology since it has wound healer, anti-aging, anti-sebum, anti-acne and moisturizing properties.

Chapter 6 - Rubber seed oil is considered as second-generation feedstock that could play a crucial role in many applications including biofuel, bio-lubricant, detergent, paints and coating, etc. This chapter will provide an overview from properties to applications of the rubber seed oil. Some of the authors' research achievement relating to application of the rubber seed oil in biodiesel synthesis will be also described.

In: Seed Oil
Editor: Nguyen Khanh Dieu Hong
ISBN: 978-1-53613-560-2

Chapter 1

MORINGA OLEIFERA SEED OIL: PRODUCTION, USES AND HEALTH BENEFITS

Silia Boukandoul[1,2], Susana Casal[2,*] and Farid Zaidi[1]

[1]Département des Sciences Alimentaires, Faculté des Sciences de la Nature et de la Vie, Université de Bejaia, Bejaia, Algeria

[2]LAQV@REQUIMTE/Laboratory of Bromatology and Hydrology, Faculty of Pharmacy, Porto University, Porto, Portugal

ABSTRACT

During the last few decades, *Moringa oleifera* seeds have gained enormous scientific attention. Indeed, the rapid growth of this tree, even under hard climatic conditions, its low demand for soil nutrients and watering, associated with its high production of seeds (more than one harvest a year) with a high oil yield (up to 44%), makes its production and development easy and reliable for the industry as a new source of oil for edible and non-edible purposes. In the past, *Moringa oleifera* seed oil was used mostly in the dermocosmetic field, including in perfumes, skin

---

* Corresponding author: sucasal@ff.up.pt.

lotions and ointments to treat disorders and damages imposed by the extremes of desert weather conditions. Scientifics evidences of its good quality and suitability for edible purposes came latter, with a particular interest on its high mono-unsaturated to saturated fatty acids ratio, included in the category of natural high oleic oils, as olive oil, and therefore desirable in terms of nutrition, health and even technological applications. It is also rich in micronutrients such as tocopherols and phytosterols, which have demonstrated strong *in vivo* antioxidant activity, and are beneficial in the prevention and treatment of several medical disorders and ailments

In this regards, a review regrouping the most pertinent information on Moringa tree propagation, as well as the composition, production, uses and health benefits of its seed oil, would be of a great interests and advantageous for further investigations and curious readers.

Keywords: *Moringa oleifera*, tree cultivation, production, seed oil, oleic acid, health benefits, oxidative stability

INTRODUCTION

Moringa oleifera Lam. (synonym: *Moringa pterygosperma* Gaertner), a member of the Moringaceae family, is one of the world's most useful trees, since almost all of its parts can be used for nutritional, medicinal or industrial purposes (Khalafalla et al., 2010) (Figure 1).

Its ability to tolerate severe environmental conditions, including drought, together with an easy propagation and adaptation to different soils (Foidl et al., 2001), has contributed for a generalised spread from its origin, in the Sub-Himalayan tracts of North-Western India, Pakistan, Bangladesh and Afghanistan (Makkar and Becker, 1997), to other tropical and sub-tropical countries, from Asia and Africa to Central America (Adejumo et al., 2013). India is the largest producer, with an annual production of 1.1 to 1.3 million tons of tender fruits from an area of 380 km^2 (Mridha, 2015).

Moringa leaves are rich in protein of high biological value, pro-vitamin A, vitamin C, minerals (particularly calcium, potassium and iron), as well as several natural antioxidants, being used as an important vegetable food due both to its nutritional properties and potential health benefits (Leone et al., 2015; Amjad et al., 2015).The fresh green pods can be eaten after boiling, but its seeds, obtained after maturation and drying, are probably the most useful part of this plant, as will be demonstrated in this chapter, mostly due to its substantial percentage of high quality oil (up to 44%) (Anwar and Bhanger, 2003; Compaoré et al., 2011; Warra, 2014).

The discovery of new sources of edible oil is highly pursued to reduce the worldwide gap between supply and demand. Considering the extremely fast and extensive growth of Moringa tree in tropical and subtropical regions of Asia and Africa (Price, 2000; Anwar and Bhanger, 2003), where malnutrition and poverty are pronounced, there has been a keen interest in the oil extracted from *M. oleifera* seeds as a new source of edible oil to be exploited (Abdulkarim et al., 2006).

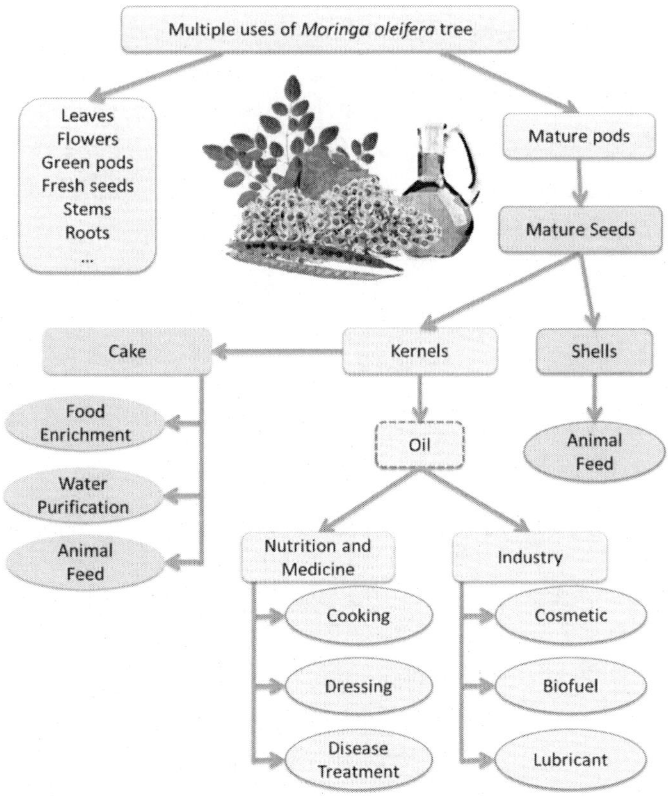

Figure 1. Multiple uses of Moringa tree.

M. oleifera oil, also known as "Ben" or "Behen" oil, is extracted from *M. oleifera* seeds kernels, presents a light yellow colour and characteristics odour, similar to that of peanut oil. The recognition of *M. oleifera* oil cosmetic value, together with its long use in traditional medicine and suitability for human consumption, have increased its cultivation interests for both edible and non-edible purposes (Foidl et al., 2001), with potential good incomes and job opportunities. The oil contains a huge percentage of oleic acid, resembling olive oil, and it is also rich in minor components such as vitamin E and phytosterols, altogether contributing to the oil's excellent oxidative stability and capacity to reduce the risk of developing coronary heart disease, among others reported health effects (Tsaknis et al., 1999; Lalas and Tsaknis, 2002; Tsaknis and Lalas, 2002; Abdulkarim et al., 2005; Abdulkarim et al., 2007; Anwar et al., 2007; Rahman et al., 2009).

Despite the considerable research interest received by *M. oleifera* oil in the last decades, there are only few published reviews. In this chapter we will summarise the most important results on *M. oleifera* oil, from its propagation and cultivation, passing by the technological processes used to extract the oil, its domestic and industrial uses, and finishing with the most important health effects, in order to provide a reliable review source for interested readers and a motivation insight for further investigations.

CLIMATE AND CULTIVATION CONDITIONS

Based on climate records, *M. oleifera* is a drought-tolerant plant that can thrive in diverse soils and in versatile conditions including hot, humid, dry tropical and subtropical regions (Ramachandran et al., 1980; Price, 2000). It tolerates a range rainfalls of 250-1500 mm per year, a wide range of pH (5-9), with an ideal temperature range of 25-35°C but tolerant to temperatures up to 40°C (Price, 2000). It grows better in loamy sand soils but its roots get rotten under excessive water (Ramachandran et al., 1980; Price, 2000; Nouman et al., 2014).

M. oleifera tree cultivation can be achieved by different methods, including direct seeding (also known as sowing), stem cuttings, and transplantation (Ramachandran et al., 1980; Price et al., 2000; Palada and Chang, 2003). The method's choice is associated to several parameters. Direct seeding is usually preferred when seeds availability in not a problem but labour is limited, while stem cuttings method is adopted when there is seed shortage but labour is plentiful (Palada and Chang, 2003). The choice is also related to the main purpose expected for the plantation: sowing is preferred for seed production while stem cuttings is usually associated to the production of leaves. Direct seeding is normally preferred to the use of stem cuttings because of its higher germination rate (Ramachandran et al., 1980; Leone at al., 2015). *M. oleifera* seeds don't have a dormancy period and can be sown as soon as they are harvested, and are expected to germinate within 1 to 2 weeks after sowing (Thurber and Fahey, 2009; Price, 2000; Ramesh-kumar et al., 2014). Transplantation is the less common, since extreme care has to be taken with young plants due to roots tenderness (Aslam et al., 2005; Gopalakrishnan et al., 2016).

Trees grown from sowing are usually more easier to maintain due to the characteristic deep tap root system developed (Price, 2000), which penetrates deep into the soil to search for water and nutrients, contributing for Moringa tree resistance to adverse climatic conditions such as drought and wind (Nouman et al., 2014).

Many studies agreed that the best period for *M. oleifera* seeds propagation is during the rainy season (Gadzirayi et al., 2013; Ramesh-Kumar et al., 2014), when the seeds can germinate and grow without any irrigation system. But for commercial purposes, seeds might also be produced during the dry season, as long as balanced irrigation is practiced (Leone et al., 2016). A study conducted by Muhl et al. (2013) showed that moderate water stress prior to floral stage stimulates flower initiation, while ample irrigation thereafter ensures good pollination, better fruit set and greater seeds yield. Furthermore, for a field establishment of *M. oleifera* as a fodder plant, Ojoawo et al. (2014) pointed out that the seed yield increases with the decrease in spacing during plantation (0.6 m x 0.6 m), while spacing of 0.9 m x 0.9 m results into larger seeds size, improving germination and growth, with consequently higher yields. The use of organic manures to enhance soil fertility has also been tested, with increase vegetative growth of *M. oleifera* seedling with poultry droppings (Adegun and Ayodele, 2013; Dania et al., 2014).

Flowers and pods are usually produced only during the second year of growth (Saint-Sauveur, 2001), and therefore the seeds yield is generally low in the first two years, but from the third year forward a single tree can yield 600 to 1600 fruits annually (Morton, 1991; Ramachandran et al., 1980). However, Ramesh-Kumar et al. (2014) stated that the seeds might be ready for harvesting nine months after sowing, and one acre yields 100 kg seeds per year. *M. oleifera* has traditionally been grown in small plantations (< 1 hectare). Only recently, some authors performed a wide range of studies on the effect of different varieties and plant density on seeds and oil yields (Ayerza et al., 2011, 2012).

Ripening time of *M. oleifera* seeds is usually related to the climatic conditions of the plantation region. Tender fruits are usually harvested during summer, but sometimes there are two crops a year, in July to September and in March to April (Ramachandran et al., 1980; Morton, 1991). *M. oleifera* seeds can be harvested by pruning the mature pods from the tree branches (Gadzirayi et al., 2013).

Oil Production and Extraction Methods

In view of *M. oleifera* tree potential for seed oil production, its high yield (32-44%) is a determinant factor, being within the reported for sunflower, canola, and palm, of 30 to 50% crude oil, and clearly higher than soybean (18-20%), the leading source of edible oil during several years (O'Brien, 2009; Nadeem and Imran, 2016). Additionally, the consistency of seeds and oil yield production from year to year is also an interesting attribute (Ayerza, 2011; Boukandoul et al., 2017). Still, the oil content of the seeds might present slight variations, due to numerous factors such as plant cultivar, soil type and available nutriments, climatic conditions, season and time of harvest, type of pre-treatment of the seeds and the type of the extraction method itself (Shahidi and Wanasundra, 2002; Ayerza, 2012).

Regarding oil extraction, cold pressing and solvent extractions have been the most traditionally used methods. However, researchers are investigating traditional and innovative, solvent and green extractive methods on *M. oleifera* seeds to find out their efficiency and profitability, while granting the use of this oil for human consumption. These methods include aqueous enzymatic extraction, and supercritical carbon dioxide extraction, as will be detailed below.

Cold pressing, known for several hundred years, is especially used to obtain high quality oils such as extra virgin olive oil and virgin rapeseed oil (Matthaus, 2012). It has also been used to obtain Moringa seed oil, but the oil yield is comparatively low (25-26%) (Tsaknis et al., 1999; Lalas and Tsaknis, 2002; Janaki and Yamuna, 2015).

Solvent extraction technique using Soxhlet-type apparatus is an effective and simple method for extraction of the seeds oil, with remarkable yields, being the most widely used, as with other oilseeds. Several processing parameters have been studied recently, as the effect of particle size (Eman and Muhamad, 2016), organic solvent type and ratio, temperature and contact time (Ghazali and Yasin, 2016; Bhutada et al., 2016). Solvent extraction of *M. oleifera* seeds oil gives the highest yield compared to other methods (Tsaknis et al., 1999; Abdulkarim et al., al., 2005; Da-Porto et al., 2016).

Supercritical carbon dioxide (SC-CO_2) extraction is currently being used to extract oil from *M. oleifera* seeds as a greener alternative to solvent extraction. Zhao and Zhang (2013) investigated the effects of extraction pressure, CO_2 flow rate, temperature, and extraction time on the yield of *M. oleifera* seed oil. Another study was conducted by Ruttarattanamongkol et al. (2014) on the yield, physico-chemical properties and chemical composition of *M. oleifera* seed oil. Generally, although a lower yield is obtained with SC-CO_2 extraction when compared to solvent extraction, the quality of the extracted oil is high (Da-Porto et al., 2016). CO_2 flow rate and temperature are important critical parameters of this method, with higher yield at 35 MPa/30°C. However, the oil extracted under these conditions is less stable to oxidation, probably due to secondary effects derived from extraction pressure and temperature effects on the fatty acids composition or other minor antioxidant compounds (Ruttarattanamongkol and Petrasch, 2016).

Aqueous enzymatic extraction is environmentally advantageous since it includes the use of water. *M. oleifera* seeds are characterised by the presence of protein as a major component (Ogunsina et al., 2010), which surround the oil droplets, being the reason why enzymes can be potentially employed for the extraction of *M. oleifera* oil from the seeds. Under the same reason, neutrase seems to be the most effective enzymes on the oil yield during aqueous enzymatic extraction (Abdulkarim et al., 2005; Abdulkarim et al., 2006; Yussof et al., 2016). Although the obtained oil yield is low, its quality is high, being less coloured and with a better oxidative stability (Yussof et al., 2016; Abdulkarim et al., 2006). However, the formation of oil in water emulsions needs a separation step to increase oil recovery (Abdulkarim et al., 2006; Abdulkarim et al., 2005, Latif et al., 2011). Also, the enzymes cost is high, making their use in large production scale critical, while the free fatty acids might increase due to enzyme activity over the fatty acids, requiring an additional neutralisation step.

Generally, most solvents are non-selective and extract also non-fat materials. Some are regarded as protective, such as antioxidants and pigments, or contribute to the typical yellow colour, as carotenoids (Abdulkarim et al., 2005). These contribute for the good physicochemical properties and stability of the seed oil without requiring additional processing operations (Tsaknis et al., 1999; Anwar and Bhanger, 2003; Abdulkarim et al., 2005; Boukandoul et al., 2017). However, others might require removal for improved performance, as is the case of gums, inducing cloudiness and reducing the oil smoke-point (Tsaknis et al., 1998, 1999). Lalas and Tsaknis (2002) correlated the amount of gums with the polarity of the solvents, with the highest amounts in oil extracted with chloroform: methanol mixture (7.2%) followed by cold pressure (2.5%) and n-hexane (0.7%). Sanchez-Machado et al. (2015) demonstrated that a simple degumming step with hot water can improve the already good edible quality of *M. oleifera* seed oil.

Assembled data shows that while the different extraction methods and additional processing steps might influence the extraction of non-fatty acids components, potentially influencing the oil performance, the fatty acid composition of *M. oleifera* seed oil is generally unaffected by the extraction method (Abdulkarim et al., 2006; Ogunsina et al., 2014; Emran and Muhamad, 2016), supporting the possibility of using any available method to extract the same high quality *M. oleifera* seed oil (Emran and Muhamad, 2016), with a strong possibility of being used without any pre-processing (refining, bleaching and deodorisation) (Abdulkarim et al., 2006), as is common in other vegetable oils, lowering the processing costs and preserving the oil natural bioactivity. Also, although lipids are usually extracted from the seed kernels, its direct extraction from whole seeds has proved to be feasible, giving an oil quality similar to the obtained from kernels alone (Boukandoul et al., 2017).

MORINGA OLEIFERA SEED OIL COMPOSITION

M. oleifera seed oil is characterised by a high mono-unsaturated to saturated fatty acids ratio, mainly due to oleic acid (up to 82%), being therefore classified as a natural high-oleic oil, similarly to olive oil. However, its fatty acid composition differs from that of olive oil in terms of linoleic acid, which is higher in olive oil, and behenic acid which is higher in *M. oleifera* seed oil (Tsaknis et al., 1999; Dollah et al., 2014). It is also a good source of natural antioxidants such as tocopherols, phytosterols, phenolic compounds and carotenoids that contribute to its unique resistance to oxidation during long storage and demanding applications (Tsaknis et al., 1998; Tsaknis et al., 1999; Lalas and Tsaknis, 2002; Anwar and Bhanger, 2003; Abdulkarim et al., 2005; Abdulkarim et al., 2007; Anwar et al., 2007; Nzikou et al., 2009; Rahman et al., 2009; Bhantagar and Gopalakrishna, 2013; Bouanga-Kalou et al., 2014; Boukandoul et al., 2017).

Table 1 represents a compilation of Moringa kernel oil yield and composition from several regions worldwide. The variation in the fat content, from 23 to 44%, is mostly a consequence of the different extraction methods, as previously discussed. Data on Moringa seed oil from Nigeria are also available, with 41.5% oil content, but no other collected characteristics were found (Ogbunugafor et al., 2011).

When the compositional parameters are compared, a high consistency is observed, as is the case of the fatty acid and triacylglycerol composition and the sterol fraction. All the oils showed the characteristic dominance of monounsaturated fatty acids, mainly oleic, followed by saturated and only traces of polyunsaturated fatty acids. Olein triglyceride fraction, confirming the dominance of oleic acid, was only detailed for Malaysian and Algerian oils varieties, being also consistent (36.7-43.0%). The sterol fraction is rich in β-sitosterol, but this oil is particularly rich in Δ^5-avenasterol, known to have anti-polymerisation activity in heated oils (Blekas et al., 2011). A focus on the total sterol amounts is also mandatory, despite being found only for some countries, with values around 5000 mg/kg (Boukandoul et al., 2017), which is very high in comparison with other vegetable oil sources.

However, when the quality parameters are compared, the variations are higher, demonstrating that the final oil quality can diverge, probably depending on the seeds characteristics, the extraction and preservation approaches. *M. oleifera* seed oil has generally low acidity. The variations observed for free fatty acid content (% oleic acid) in Table 1 can be again induced by the different extraction methods, imposed by water contact and enzymatic activity. Also, different oxidation degrees can be deduced from the K_{232} and K_{270} values, together with the tocopherol content, also highly variable. While the former demonstrates the presence of primary and secondary oxidation products, tocopherol reduction should be a consequent of its antioxidant activity, being consumed to protect the oil matrix. This could be the case of the Indian oils and some of the Kenyan ones, simultaneously with high K_{232} and K_{270} values and low tocopherol content.

Table 1. Oil content, stability parameters and essential constituents of *M. oleifera* seed oil from different regions around the world*

Parameters	Algeria [A]	Bangla-desh [B]	Brazil [C]	Burkina Faso [D]	Congo [E]	Cuba [F]	India [G]	Kenya [H]	Malawi [I]	Mala-ysia [J]	Pakis-tan [K]	Overall range
Fat content (%)	37.0 – 37.4	35.6 – 40.2	39.0	43.6	38.5 – 40.0	24.1 – 26.5	24.2 – 39.4	25.1 – 41.4	26.3 – 35.5	22.6 – 31.0	30.4 – 42.0	22.6 – 43.6
Acidity (% oleic acid)	0.9 – 1.0	0.7 – 1.1	4.0	NR	1.1 – 2.1	NR	3.5 – 4.0	0.9 – 1.9	0.8 – 1.2	0.2 – 2.5	0.3 – 0.8	0.2 – 4.0
K232	1.45– 1.86	1.85 – 2.28	NR	NR	NR	NR	NR	1.16 – 3.15	1.19 – 1.44	1.36	1.40 – 1.98	1.16 – 3.15
K270	0.16 – 0.24	0.44 – 0.92	NR	NR	NR	NR	NR	0.19 – 1.13	0.12 – 0.16	0.05	0.18 – 1.02	0.05 – 1.13
Induction period (h) (120ºC)	42.1 – 56.6	11.7 – 54.1	NR	NR	NR	NR	NR	28.2 – 46.2 (8.7 – 18.9)	68.4 – 123 (23.7 – 34.7)	NR	9.6 – 10.3 (8.3 – 9.6)	8.3 – 123
Oleic acid (%)	71.0 – 71.7	71.3 – 74.4	74.8 – 78.0	72.4	74.4 – 74.9	73.1 – 77.5	78.7 – 79.5	71.2 – 75.4	67.7 – 67.8	67.9 – 81.7	72.0 – 78.6	67.7 – 81.7
Behenic acid (%)	6.1 – 6.8	6.2 – 6.6	4.0 - 5.6	6.95	5.2 – 5.3	5.2 – 5.8	4.5 – 5.1	5.8 – 6.7	6.7 – 6.8	4.9 – 6.2	3.7 – 7.0	3.7 – 7.0
SFA (%)	22.0 – 23.7	21.9 – 23.6	19.0 – 21.5	21.6	20.4	16.9 – 21.3	17.2 – 18.3	19.1 – 23.8	22.7 – 23.1	15.8 – 27.0	16.9 – 24.7	15.8 – 27.0
MUFA (%)	74.9 – 76.2	75.0 – 77.8	78.1 – 80.0	76.5	78.5 – 78.9	77.6 – 78.5	79.9 – 80.7	75.0 – 80.2	71.5 – 71.7	71.6 – 84.2	74.5 – 81.6	71.5 – 84.2
PUFA (%)	0.9 – 1.21	0.5 – 1.2	0.4 – 1	1.4	0.7 – 1.0	0.3 – 1.14	1.8 – 2.2	0.2 – 1.0	0.9 – 1.0	0.7 – 1.3	0.3 – 1.9	0.2 – 2.2

Parameters	Algeria [A]	Bangla-desh [B]	Brazil [C]	Burkina Faso [D]	Congo [E]	Cuba [F]	India [G]	Kenya [H]	Malawi [I]	Mala-ysia [J]	Pakis-tan [K]	Overall range
Total tocopherols (mg/kg)	301 – 325	241 – 294	NR	NR	NR	NR	88 – 96	21 – 217	255 – 515	NR	238 – 321 (214 – 244)	21 – 515
β- Sitosterol (%)	45.3 – 48.2	46.2 – 47.9	NR	NR	NR	NR	NR	43.7 – 50.1	46.7 – 47.1	NR	42.6 – 52.2	42.6 – 52.2
Δ5-Avenasterol (%)	9.2 – 13.7	6.1 – 9.8	NR	NR	NR	NR	NR	8.5 – 12.8	1.2 – 3.0	NR	8.9 – 12.0	1.2-13.7

Literature: [A]: Boukandoul et al., 2017. [B]: Rahman et al., 2009. [C]: Da Silva et al., 2010; Pereira et al., 2016. [D]: Compaoré et al., 2011. [E]: Nzikou et al., 2009; Bouanga-Kalou et al., 2014. [F]: Martin et al., 2010; Delange et al., 2014. [G]: Bhantagar and Gopala khrishna, 2013; Ogunsina et al., 2014. [H]: Tsaknis et al., 1999; Lalas and Tsaknis, 2002. [I]: Tsaknis et al., 1998. [J]: Mohammed et al., 2003; Abdulkarim et al., 2005; Abdulkarim et al., 2007; Dollah et al., 2014. [K]: Anwar and Bhanger, 2003; Anwar et al., 2005; Anwar et al., 2006; Anwar et al., 2007; Anwar and Rashid, 2007. NR: not reported.

The induction period is probably the clearer reflect of Moringa oil excellent stability, and the influence of the minor compounds on the oil characteristics. For the highest quality Moringa oils the induction period ranged between 40 to 50 hours, but values up to 123 h have been found (Table1), demonstrating its capacity to resist to oxidation for long periods, a characteristic that is interesting both for cooking and industrial purposes. These values are higher than those presented by the majority of edible vegetable oils, olive oil included. Aware that the fatty acid composition is rather constant between Moringa seed oils, even from diverse origins, the minor compounds present in the oil should have a strong influence on the oil behaviour, including vitamin E, sterols, carotenoids and phenolic compounds. This justifies the decrease on the stability found after refining, where some of these compound are partially eliminated, together with gums, where phosphatides, proteins and colloidal substances are included (Tsaknis et al, 1998).This is particularly evident for one of the samples from Malawi, extracted with chloroform: methanol, with the induction period being reduced from 123 h to just 31.8 h after degumming. However, water degumming is essential when the oils are intended for thermal purposes, including frying, increasing its performance.

MORINGA OLEIFERA SEED OIL USES

M. oleifera seed oil knows numerous uses: it is used as dressing, for cooking, for fine machine lubrication, in the manufacture of perfumes, skin and hair care products, and in several industrial as well as medical products (Tsaknis et al., 1998; Foidl et al., 2001).

M. oleifera seed oil found application since ancient times when the Romans, Greeks and Egyptians started extracting oil from the seeds and used it for perfume and skin lotions and ointments, due to its great power to absorb and retain volatile substances. Interestingly, and still far from scientific evidences, it was used as a potent cure for skin disorders caused by harsh climatic conditions, which makes it an ideal moisturiser, healing and soothing emollient for rough, dry skin and therapeutic massages. In the

19th century, West Indies exported Moringa oil to Europe for perfumes industries (Foidl et al., 2001; Warra, 2014). *M. oleifera* oil has also been shown to be particularly effective in the manufacture of soap, producing a stable lather with high washing efficiency (Warra, 2007). It is also considered to have relative potential for cosmetics, like the African shea butter, such as in lip balms and creams (Warra, 2014). More recently, it began to be also widely used for the production of biodiesel, with a higher octane number (Rashid et al., 2008; Da-Silva et al., 2010).

Scientific curiosity has also driven research into the demonstration of its suitability for human consumption (Tsaknis et al., 1998; Tsaknis et al., 1999; Anwar and Bhanger, 2003; Abdulkarim et al., 2005), after the seeds have been found non-toxic in an earlier study conducted by Berger et al. (1984). Its high oleic acid is the strongest attribute, which makes it desirable for human consumption in terms of nutrition, health and even technological resistance for some applications such as cooking and frying. Accordingly, *M. oleifera* seed oil proved to offer higher resistance to auto-oxidation and replace synthetic antioxidants for long term conservation of butter oil at ambient temperature (Nadeem et al., 2013). Anwar et al. (2007) blended sunflower, canola and soybean oils with *M. oleifera* seed oil, at various concentrations, and studied some oxidative parameters during long storage at room temperature, showing that *M. oleifera* oil enhanced the oxidative stability of these vegetable oils. Moreover, Abdulkarim et al. (2007) compared *M. oleifera* seed oil resistance during deep frying with some vegetable oils like canola, soybean and palm olein; *M. oleifera* oil was found to be more stable during frying applications. In another study, Dollah et al.(2014) blended *M. oleifera* seed oil with palm olein (PO), palm stearin (PS), palm kernel (PKO) and virgin coconut (VCO) oils in order to modify their physical and chemical properties, and reported several potential uses of the blends, as high oleic *trans* free fat bakery shortening formulations (MOO/PS; 50:50 and 30:70), high stable frying oil and salad dressing (MOO/PO), or high oleic liquid margarines, soft margarines and spread formulations (MOO/PKO and MOO/VCO). Moreover, *M. oleifera* seed oil can be used directly as a natural rich source of behenic acid, which has been used as an oil structuring and solidifying agent in margarine, shortening, and foods containing semi-solid and solid fats (Abdulkarim et al., 2005).

Furthermore, the remaining cake after oil extraction is characterised by high protein content (33.3-62.8%) (Oliveira et al., 1999; Ogunsina et al., 2010), from which many valorisation issues can be developed, such as enrichment and fortification of food products in order to increase the protein intake, especially in terms of methionine and cysteine (Ogunsina et al., 2011; Olagbemide and Alikwe, 2014; Oliveira et al., 1999). One more interesting application of the defatted *M. oleifera* seed is the purification of turbid water due to the ionic characteristic of its proteins, acting as a natural coagulant and flocculent, while lowering micro-organisms and bacteria levels, making it more suitable for drinking (Saint-Sauveur, 2001; Mangale et al., 2012; Gadzirayi et al., 2013). Still, further studies are required to ascertain on the impact of the ingestion of solubilised compounds, including water soluble lectins with potential hemagglutinating action (Santos et al., 2005).

Pursue for new commercial uses of Moringa oil is particularly evident by the high amount of patents registered over the years. *M. oleifera* oil is particularly patented in the cosmetic field, but most patents are associated to the use of dry *M. oleifera* leaf extracts as a functional food. Despite the great number of researches related to water purification as well as metal and heavy metal adsorption, the number of patents in these fields remains small (Dou and Kister, 2016).

HEALTH BENEFITS

Nowadays, the use of oils has known a huge increase for preventing or treating many health diseases and ailments. *M. oleifera* seed oil can be viewed as a powerful natural source of oleic acid, which has been shown to reduce serum cholesterol and low-density lipoprotein-cholesterol levels, without impacting high-density lipoprotein-cholesterol, minimising the risk of cardiovascular diseases (O'Brien, 2009). It is also reported to act as a precursor of the omega 9 fatty acids family (Nadeem and Imran, 2016).

Naturally high oleic oils, as olive oil, were found to reduce an overall risk of all-cause mortality (11%), cardiovascular mortality (12%), cardiovascular events (9%), and stroke (17%) (Schwingshacki and Hoffmann, 2014).

Despite the small levels of micro-components present in *M. oleifera* seed oil, they have been found to play a vital role in the battle against several diseases. *M. oleifera* seed oil contains natural antioxidants which are believed to mediate its hepatoprotective effects, acting efficiency against xenobiotic-induced liver disorders (Olatosin et al., 2014). There is a beneficial relationship between the antioxidant activity and the hepatoprotective effect of *M. oleifera* seed oil and substantiate its use in liver disorders by folk medicine practitioners (Al-Said et al., 2012). Tocopherols are antioxidants, functioning as a nonspecific chain-breaking antioxidant that prevents propagation of lipid oxidation (O'Brien, 2009) by stabilising hydroperoxyl and other free radicals. Different tocopherol homologues show different antioxidant activities in model systems, both *in vivo* and *in vitro*; α- and γ-tocopherols being the strongest antioxidants in food systems (Tsao and Li, 2008; O'Brien, 2009). Moreover, α-tocopherol is the most dominant in this oil with representative values (up to 515 mg/kg – Table 1). Vitamin E was found to be also effective against various diseases such as atherosclerosis, oxidative stress, cancer, coronary diseases, and diabetes, among others (Rizvi et al., 2014). Carotenoids are also shown to protect oils from photo-oxidation (O'Brien, 2009). Phytosterols, namely β-sitosterol, is shown to block the biochemical events of cholesterol formation, to lower heart disease risks and to possess anti-inflammatory effects (O'Brien, 2009; Nadeem and Imran, 2016) and anti-diabetic potential (Gupta et al. 2011). More recently, other antidiabetic components, which can serve as oral hypoglycaemic agent or adjuvant, have been reported in Moringa oil (Busari et al. 2014, 2015).

CONCLUSION

M. oleifera seeds are regarded as a potential source of oil and proteins especially in under developed countries, where Moringa plant thrives well. The oil can be used for edible and non-edible applications and the proteins for food enrichment and fortification.

Given the consistency of oil content and compositional parameters of *M. oleifera* seed oil reported for different regions, it could be considered as a valuable source high natural monounsaturated fatty acid source, together with natural antioxidants such as tocopherols and phytosterols. Moreover, its extraction can be achieved by diverse techniques, with a general good quality, disabling the need for full refining, usually restricted to neutralisation and degumming.

The scientific evidences to support the numerous health effects reported on the basis of traditional medicine is interesting several researchers worldwide, being of particular interest for the development of new medicines, while increasing the profit of this "miracle tree".

REFERENCES

Abdulkarim, S. M., Long, K., Lai, O. M., Muhammad, S. K. S., and Ghazali, H. M. 2005. "Some physico-chemical properties of *Moringa oleifera* seed oil extracted using solvent and aqueous enzymatic methods." *Food Chemistry* 93: 353-263.

Abdulkarim, S. M., Lai, O. M., Muhammad, S. K. S., Long, K., and Ghazali, H. M. 2006. "Use of enzymes to enhance oil recovery during aqueous extraction of *Moringa oleifera* seeds oil." *Journal of Food Lipids* 13: 113-130.

Abdulkarim, S. M., Long, K., Lai, O. M., Muhammad, S. K. S., and Ghazali, H. M. 2007. "Frying quality and stability of high oleic *Moringa oleifera* seed oil in comparison with other vegetable oils. *Food Chemistry."* 105: 1382-1389.

Adegun, M. K. and Ayodele, O. J. 2015. "Growth and yield of *Moringa oleifera* as influenced by spacing and organic manures in South-Western Nigeria."*International Journal of Agronomy and Agricultural Research* 6: 30-37.

Adejumo, B. A., Alakowe, A. T. and Obi, D. 2013. "Effect of Heat Treatment on the Characteristics and Oil Yield of *Moringa oleifera* Seeds." *International Journal of Engineering and Science* 2: 232-239.

Al-Said, M. S., Mothana, R. A., Al-Yahya, M. A., Al-Blowi, A. S., Al-Sohaibani, M., Ahmed, A. F. and Rafatullah, S. 2012. "Edible oils for liver protection: Hepatoprotective potentiality of *Moringa oleifera* seed oil against chemical-induced hepatitis in rats." *Journal of Food science* 77 (7): T124-T130.

Amjad, M. Sh., Qureshi, H., Arshad, M., Chaudhari, S. Kh. and Masood, M. 2015. "The incredible queen of green: Nutritive value and therapeutic potential of *Moringa oleifera* Lam." *Journal of Coastal Life Medicine*, 3 (9): 744-751.

Anwar, F., and Bhanger, M. I. 2003. "Analytical characterization of *Moringa oleifera* seed oil grown in temperate regions of Pakistan." *Journal of Agricultural and Food Chemistry* 51: 6558-6563.

Anwar, F., Ashraf, M. and Bhanger, M. I. 2005. "Interprovenance variation in the composition of *Moringa oleifera* oilseeds from Pakistan."*Journal of the American Oil Chemist's Society* 82 (1): 45-51.

Anwar, F., Zafar, S. N. and Rashid, U. 2006. "Characterization of *Moringa oleifera* seed oil from drought and irrigated regions of Punjab, Pakistan."*Grasas y Aceites* 57 (2): 160-168.

Anwar, F., Hussain, A. I., Iqbal, S. and Bhanger, M. I. 2007. "Enhancement of the oxidative stability of some vegetable oils by blending with *Moringa oleifera* oil." *Food Chemistry* 103: 1181-1191.

Anwar, F. and Rashid, U. 2007. "Physico-chemical characteristics of *Moringa oleifera* seeds and seeds oil from a wild provenance of Pakistan."*Pakistan Journal of Botany* 39 (5): 1443-1453.

Aslam, M. F., Anwar, R., Nadeem, U., Rashid, T. G., Kazi, A. and Nadeem, M. 2005. "Mineral composition of *Moringa oleifera* leaves and pods from different regions of Punjab, Pakistan." *Asian Journal of Plant Science* 4: 417-421.

Ayerza, R. 2011. "Seed yield components, oil content, and fatty acid composition of two cultivars of moringa (*Moringa oleifera* Lam.) growing in the Arid Chaco of Argentina." *Industrial Crops and Products* 33: 389-394.

Ayerza, R. 2012. "Seed and oil yields of *Moringa oleifera* variety Periyakalum-1 introduced for oil production in four ecosystems of South America."*Industrial Crops and Products* 36: 70–73.

Berger, M.R., Habs, M., Jahn, S.A.A. and Schmahl, A. 1984. "Toxicological assessment of seeds from *Moringa oleifera* and *Moringa stenopetala*, two highly efficient primary coagulants for domestic water treatment of tropical raw waters." *East African Medical Journal* 61: 712-716.

Bhatnagar, A. S., Gopala Krishna, A. G. 2013. "Natural antioxidant of Jaffna variety of *Moringa oleifera* seed oil from Indian origin as compared to other vegetable oils." *Grasas y Aceites* 64: 537-545.

Bhutada, P. R., Jadhav, A. J., Pinjari, D. V. and Nemade, P. R. 2016. "Solvent assisted extraction of *Moringa oleifera* Lam. seeds."*Industrial Crops and Products* 88: 74-80.

Blekas, G., Bouskou, D. 2011. "Phytosterols and frying oils." In: Bouskou, D., Elmadfa, I. (Eds.), *Frying of Food: Oxidation, Nutrient and non-Nutrient Antioxidants, Biologically Active Compounds, and High Temperatures*, CRC Press, New York, 225-232.

Bouanga-Kalou, S., Dhellot, J. R., Matos, L., Kimbonguila, A., Mountou-Tchitoula, D., Malela, K. E., Hpunpunpu, C. H., Nzikou, J. M., Silou, and Th., Desobry, S. 2014. "Characteristic physicochemical of oil extract from *Moringa oleifera* and the kinetics of degradation of the oil during heating." *Research Journal of Applied Sciences and Engineering Technology* 7: 3649-3655.

Boukandoul, S., Casal, S., Cruz, R. Pinto, C. and Zaidi, F. 2017. "Algerian *Moringa oleifera* whole seeds and kernels oils: characterization, oxidative stability and antioxidant capacity." *European Journal of Lipid Science and Technology* 118: doi: 10.1002/ejlt.201600410.

Busari, M. B., Muhammad H. L., Ogbadoyi, E. O., Abdulrasheed-Adeleke, T. and Sani, S. 2014. "Hypoglycaemic properties of *Moringa oleifera* Lam seeds oil in normoglycaemic rats." *Journal of Pharmacy and Biological Sciences* 9 (6): 23-27.

Busari, M. B., Muhammad H. L., Ogbadoyi, E. O., Kabiru, A. Y., Sani, S. and Yusuf, R. S. 2015. "In vivo evaluation of antidiabetic properties of seed oil of *Moringa oleifera* Lam." *Journal of Applied Life Sciences Internat*ional 2 (4): 160-174.

Compaoré, W. R., Nikièma, P. A., Bassolé, H. I. N., Savadogo, A., Mouecoucou, J., Hounhouigan, D. J. and Traoré, S. A. 2011. "Chemical composition and antioxidative properties of seeds of *Moringa oleifera* and pulps of *Parkia biglobosa* and *Adansonia digitata* commonly used in food fortification in Burkina Faso." *Current Research Journal of Biological Sciences* 3 (1): 64-72.

Dania, S. O., Akpansubi, P. and Eghagara, O. O. 2014. "Comparative effects of different fertilizer sources on the growth and nutrient content of Moringa (*Moringa oleifera*) seedling in Greenhouse Trial." *Hinhawi Publishing Corporation Advances in Agriculture* 2014: 1-6.

Da-Porto, C., Decorti, D. and Natolino, A. 2016. "Microwave pretreatment of *Moringa oleifera* seed: Effect on oil obtained by pilot-scale supercritical carbon dioxide extraction and Soxhlet apparatus." *Journal of Supercritical Fluids* 107: 38-43.

Da-Silva, J. P.V., Serra, T. M., Gossmann, M. Wolf, C. R., Meneghetti, M. R. and Meneghetti, S. M. P. 2010. "*Moringa oleifera* oil: Studies of characterization and biodiesel production." *Biomass and Bioenergy* 34: 1527-1530.

Delange, D. M., Murillo, R. V., Gonzalez Canavaciodo, V. L. and Amaro, J. G. 2014. "Fatty acid composition from seed oil from *Moringa oleifera* grown in Havana, Cuba." *Revista Cubana de Plantas Medicinales* 19: 197-204.

Dollah, S., Abdulkarim, S. M., Ahmad, S. H., Khoramnia, A., Ghazali, H. M. 2014."Physical properties and potential food applications of *Moringa oleifera* seed oil blended with other vegetable oils." *Journal of Oleo Science* 63: 811-822.

Dou, H. and Kister, J. 2016. "Research and development on *Moringa oleifera* – Comparison between academic research and patents." *World Patent Information* 47: 21-33.

Emran, N. A. and Muhamed, N. S. 2016. "Comparison of *Moringa oleifera* seeds oil characterization produced chemically and mechanically."*International Conference on Chemical Engineering and Bioprocess Engineering*: *Earth and Environmental Science* 36. doi: 10.1088/1755-1315/36/1/012063.

Foidl N, Makkar H. P. S., Becker K. 2001. "The potential of *Moringa oleifera* for agricultural and industrial uses." In: *Proceedings of the International Workshop "What development potential for Moringa products",* Dares-Salaam, Tanzania, 47-67.

Gadzirayi, C. T., Mudyiwa1, S. M., Mupangwa J. F., and Gotosa, J. 2013. "Cultivation Practices and Utilization of *Moringa oleifera* Provenances by Small Holder Farmers: Case of Zimbabwe." *Asian Journal of Agricultural Extension, Economics and Sociology* 2 (2): 152-162.

Ghazali, Q. and Yasin, N. H. M. 2016. "The effect of organic solvent, temperature and mixing time on the production of oil from *Moringa oleifera* seeds." International Conference on Chemical Engineering and Bioprocess Engineering: *Earth and Environmental Science*, 36 doi: 10.1088/1755-1315/36/1/012053.

Gopalakrishnan, L., Doriya, K. and Kumar, D. S. 2016. "*Moringa oleifera*: A review on nutritive importance and its medical application." *Food Science and Human Wellness* 5: 49-56.

Gupta, R., Sharma, A. K.; Dobhal, M. P., Sharma, M. C., Gupta, R.S. 2011. "Antidiabetic and antioxidant potential of β-sitosterol in streptozotocin-induced experimental hyperglycemia." *Journal of Diabetes* 3: 29-37.

Janaki, S. and Yamuna, D. P. 2015. "Extraction of cold press Moringa oil." *International Journal of current Research* 7 (4): 14956-14957.

Khalafalla, M. M., Abdellatef, E., Dafalla, H. M., Nassrallah, A. A., Aboul-Enein, Kh. M., Lightfoot, D. A., El-Deeb, F. E. and El-Shemy, H. A. 2010. "Active principle from *Moringa oleifera* Lam leaves effective against two leukemias and a hepatocarcinoma." *African Journal of Biotechnology*, 9 (49): 8467-8471.

Lalas, S., Tsaknis, J. 2002. "Extraction and identification of natural antioxidant from the seeds of the *Moringa oleifera* tree variety of Malawi." *Journal of American Oil Chemists Society* 79: 677-683.

Latif, S., Anwar, F., Hussain, A. I. and Shahid, M. 2011. "Aqueous enzymatic process for oil and protein extraction from *Moringa oleifera* seed." *European Journal of Lipid Science and Technology* 113: 1012-1018.

Leone, A., Spada, A., Battezzati, A., Schiraldi, A., Aristil, J. and Bertoli, S. 2015. "Cultivation, Genetic, Ethnopharmacology, Phytochemistry and Pharmacology of *Moringa oleifera* Leaves: An Overview." *International Journal of Molecular Sciences* 16: 12791-12835.

Leone, A., Spada, A., Battezzati, A., Schiraldi, A., Aristil, J. and Bertoli, S. 2016. "*Moringa oleifera* seeds and oil: characteristics and uses for human health." *International Journal of Molecular Sciences*, 17 (2141) doi:10.3390/ijms17122141.

Makkar H.P.S. and Becker K. 1997. "Nutrients and antiquality factors in different morphological parts of the *Moringa oleifera* tree." *Journal of Agricultural Sciences*, 128:311-332.

Mangale, S. M., Chonde, S. G., Jadhav, A. S. and Raut, P. D. 2012. "Study of *Moringa oleifera* (Drumstick) seed as natural Absorbent and Antimicrobial agent for River water treatment." *Journal of Natural Products and Plant Resources* 2 (1): 89-100.

Martin, C., Moure, A., Martin, G., Carrillo, E., Dominguez, H. and Parajo, J. C. 2010. "Fractional characteristics of jatropha, neem, moringa, trisperma, castor and candlenut seeds as potential feedstocks for biodiesel production in Cuba." *Biomass and Bioenergy* 34: 533-538.

Matthaus, B. 2012."Oil technology." *In* Gupta, S. K. (Eds.), *Technological innovations in major oil crops.* Springer Science and Business Media, 36-42.

Mohammed, A. S., Lai, O. M., Muhammad, S. K. S., Long, K. and Ghazali, H. M. 2003. "Moringa oleifera, Potentially a New Source of oleic acid-type oil for Malaysia." In: Hassan, M. A. et al. (Eds.), *Investing in Innovation,* Vol 3, Bioscience and Biotechnology, Serdang Press, Malaysia, 137-140.

Morton, J. F. 1991. "The horseradish tree, Moringa Pterygosperma (Moringaceae) – A boon to arid lands?" *Economic Botany* 45 (3): 318–333.

Mridha, M.A.U. 2015. "Prospects of Moringa cultivation in Saudi Arabia." *Journal of Applied Environmental and Biological Sciences* 5(3): 39-46.

Muhl, Q. E., Du Toit, E. S., Steyn, J. M. and Apostolides, Z. 2013. "Bud development, flowering and fruit set of *Moringa oleifera* Lam. (Horseradish Tree) as affected by various irrigation levels." *Journal of Agriculture and Rural Development in the Tropics and Subtropics* 114: 79-87.

Nadeem, M., Hussain, I. and Abdullah, M., 2013. "Improvement of oxidative stability of butter oil by blending with *Moringa oleifera* oil." *Journal of Food Processing and Preservation* 38: 1491-1500.

Nadeem, M., and Imra, M. 2016. "Promising features of *Moringa oleifera* oil: recent updates and perspectives." *Lipids in Health and Disease* 15 (212).doi: 10.1186/s12944-016-0379-0.

Nouman, W., Basra, Sh.M. A., Siddiqui, M. T., Yasmeen, A. Gull, T. and Alcayde, M. A.C. 2014. "Potential of *Moringa oleifera* L. as livestock fodder crop: a review." *Turkish Journal of Agriculture and Forestry* 38: 1-14.

Nzikou, J. M., Matos, L., Moussounga, J. E., Ndangui, C. B., Kimbonguila, A., Silou, Th., Linder, M., and Desorby, S. 2009. "Characterisation of *Moringa oleifera* seed oil variety Congo-Brazzaville." *Journal of Food Technology* 7: 59-65.

O'Brien, R. D. 2009. *Fats and Oils: Formulating and Processing for Applications*, 1-66. London (New York) CRC Press.

Ogbunugafor, H. A., Eneh, F. U., Ozumba, A. N., Igwo-Ezikpe, M. N., Okpuzor, J., Igwilo, I. O., Adenekan, S. O., Onyekwelu, O. A. 2011. "Physico-chemical and Antioxidant Properties of *Moringa oleifera* Seed Oil." *Pakistan Journal of Nutrition*10: 409-414.

Ogunsina, B.S., Radha, C. and Govardhan Singh, R.S. 2010. "Physicochemical and functional properties of full-fat and defatted *Moringa oleifera* kernel flour." *International Journal of Food Science and Technology* 45: 2433-2439.

Ogunsina, B.S., Radha, C. and Indrani, D. 2011. "Quality characteristics of bread and cookies enriched with debittered *Moringa oleifera* seed flour." *International of Food Sciences and Nutrition* 62 (2): 185-194.

Ogunsina, B. S., Indira, T. N., Bhatnagar, A. S., Radha, C., Debnath, S., Gopala Krishna, A. G. 2014. "Quality characteristics and stability of *Moringa oleifera* seed oil of Indian origin." *Journal of Food Science and Technology* 51: 503-510.

Ojoawo, O. T., Akinlade, J. A., Akingbade, A. A. and Aderinola, O. A. 2014. "Influence of planting distance on seed yield and size of *Moringa oleifera*." *International Journal of Research in Agricultural Sciences* 1 (5): 2348-3997.

Olagbemide, P. T. and Alikwe, P.C.N. 2014. "Proximate analysis and chemical composition of raw and defatted *Moringa oleifera* kernel." *Advances in Life Science and Technology* 24: 92-99.

Olatosin, T. M., Akinduko, D. S., Uche, C. Z. and Bardi, J. 2014. "Effects of *Moringa oleifera* seed oil on acetaminophen-induced oxidative stress and liver damage in wistar albino rats." *Journal of Pharmacy and Biological Sciences* 9 (2): 53-59.

Oliveira, J.T.A., Silveira, S.B., Vasconcelos, I.M., Cavada, B.S. and Moreira, R.A. 1999. "Compositional and nutritional attributes of seeds from the multiple purpose tree *Moringa oleifera* Lamarck." *Journal of Science Food and agriculture* 79: 815-820.

Palada, M. C. and Chang, L. C. 2003. "Suggested cultural practices for Moringa." *A. V. R. D. C. Pub* 3: 1-5.

Pereira, F. S. G., Galvao, C. C., De Lima, V. F. da Rocha, M. F. A., Schuler, A. R. P., Da Silva, V. L. and Lima Filho, N. M. 2016. "The versatility of the *Moringa oleifera* oil in sustainable applications." *Oilseeds & fats and Lipids*. doi: 10.1051/ocl/2016027.

Price, M. L. 2000. *"The Moringa tree. Echo Technical Note."* Available at http://chenetwork.org/files_pdf/Moringa.pdf.

Rahman, I. M. M., Barua, S., Nazimuddin, M., Begum, Z. A., Rahman, M. A. and Hasegawa, H. 2009. "Physicochemical properties of *Moringa oleifera* Lam. seed oil of the indigenous-cultivar of Bangladesh." *Journal of Food Lipids* 16: 540-553.

Ramachandran, C., Peter, K. V., and Gopalakrishnan, K. (1980). Drumstick (*Moringa oleifera*): A multiple Indian vegetable. *Economic Botany*, 34 (3): 276-283.

Ramesh-Kumar, A. R., Prabhu, M., Ponnuswami, V., Lakshmanan, V. and Nithyadevi, A. 2014. "Scientific seed production techniques in Moringa." *Agricultural Reviews* 35 (1): 69-73.

Rashid, U., Anwar, F., Moser, B. R., and Knothe, G. 2008. "*Moringa oleifera* oil: A possible source of biodiesel." *Bioresource Technology* 99: 8175-8179.

Rizvi, S., Raza, S. T., Ahmed, F., Ahmad, A., Abbas, Sh. and Mahdi, F. 2014. "The role of vitamin E in human health and some diseases." *Sultan Qaboos University Med Journal* 14: 157-165.

Ruttarattanamongkol, Kh., Siebenhandl-Ehn, S., Schreiner, M., and Petrasch, A. M. 2014. "Pilot-scale supercritical carbon dioxide extraction, physico-chemical properties and profile characterization of *Moringa oleifera* seed oil in comparison with conventional extraction methods." *Industrial Crops and Products* 58: 68-77.

Ruttarattanamongkol, Kh. and Petrasch, A. 2016. "Oxidative susceptibility and thermal properties of *Moringa oleifera* seed oil obtained by pilot-scale subcritical and supercritical carbon dioxide extraction." *Journal of Food Press Engineering* 39: 226-236.

Sánchez-Machado, D. I., López-Cervantes, J., Núñez-Gastélum, J. A., de la Mora-López, G. S., López-Hernández, J. and Paseiro-Losada, P. 2015. "Effect of the refining process on *Moringa oleifera* seed oil quality." *Food Chemistry* 187: 53-57.

Saint-Sauveur, A. (de) 2001. "'Moringa exploitation in the world': State of knowledge and challenges." Development Potential for Moringa Products. *Dar es Salaam, Tanzania, International Workshop* 29 Oct. - 2 Nov.

Santos, A. F. S., Argolo, A. C. C., Coelho, L. C. B. B and Paiva, P. M. G. 2005. "Detection of water soluble lectin and antioxidant component from *Moringa oleifera* seeds." *Water Research* 39: 975-980.

Schwingshachi, L. and Hoffmann, G. 2014. "Monounsaturated fatty acids, olive oil and health status: a systematic review and meta-analysis of cohort studies." *Lipids in Health and Disease* 13 (154). doi: 10.1186/1476-511X-13-154.

Shahidi, F. and Wanasundara, P. K. J. P. D. 2002. "Extraction and analysis of lipids." In: Akoh C.C. and Min, D.B. (Eds.), *Food Lipids: Chemistry, Nutrition, and Biotechnology*, 133–168. Marcel Dekker, Inc., New York.

Thurber, M. D. and Fahey, J. W. 2009. "Adoption of *Moringa oleifera* to combat under-nutrition viewed through the lens of the "Diffusion of Innovations" theory." *Ecology of Food and Nutrition* 48 (3): 2012-225.

Tsao, R. and Li, L. 2008. "Phytochemical profiles and potential health of benefits of heart nuts (*Juglans ailanthifolia* var. Cordiformis): a comparison with the common walnut (*Juglans regia* L.)." *In*: Alasalvar, C. and Shahidi, F. (Eds.), *Tree nuts: composition, phytochemicals, and health effects*. 242-245. London, New York. CRC Press, Taylor and Francis group.

Tsaknis, J. and Lalas, S. 2002. "Stability during frying of *Moringa oleifera* seed oil variety "Periyakulam 1"." *Journal of Food Composition and Analysis* 15: 79-101.

Tsaknis, J., Lalas, S., Gergis, V. and Spiliotis, V. 1998. "A total characterisation of *Moringa oleifera* Malawi seed oil." *La Rivista Italiana Delle Sostanze Grasse* LXXV: 21-27.

Tsaknis, J., Lalas, S., Gergis, V., Douroglou, V., and Spiliotis, V. 1999. "Characterization of *Moringa oleifera* variety Mbololo seed oil of Kenya." *Journal of Agricultural Food Chemistry* 47: 4495-4499.

Warra A. A. 2007. "Production of soap from an indigenous *Moringa oleifera* Lam. seed oil." *Journal of Raw Materials and Research* 7: (1 and 2): 26-35.

Warra, A.A. 2014. "A review of *Moringa oleifera* Lam. seed oil prospects in personal care formulations." *Research and Reviews: Journal of Pharmaceutics and Nanotechnology* 2 (3): 31-34.

Yussof, M. M., Gordon, M. H., Ezeh, O. and Niranjan, K. 2016. "Aqueous enzymatic extraction of *Moringa oleifera* oil." *Food Chemistry* 211: 400-408.

Zhao, S. and Zhang, D. 2013. "A parametric study of supercritical carbon dioxide extraction of oil from *Moringa oleifera* seeds using a response surface methodology." *Separation and Purification Technology* 113: 9-17.

In: Seed Oil ISBN: 978-1-53613-560-2
Editor: Hong Nguyen Khanh Dieu

Chapter 2

NEEM SEED OIL: PRODUCTION, USES AND BENEFITS

Sunday A. Dialoke*, PhD
Depattment of Crop Science and Technology,
School of Agriculture and Agricultural Technology,
Federal University of Technology, Owerri, Imo State, Nigeria

ABSTRACT

The Agrochemicals have been conventional in the control of Agricultural pests. These are Synthetic pesticides used during crop production to control pests. They are very useful in crop production, however it has been noticed that the use of this form of pesticide has effects which are detrimental to man and his environment. On man, there are its recorded effects on the immune system, the endocrine gland as well as the reproductive tract. Some of which includes respiratory organ's malfunction, memory disorder, birth defects, miscarriages, cancer etc. Recorded effects on the environment include land, water and air pollution. In view of these problems, the exploration of ecologically safe

* Corresponding Author Email: akuamka@yahoo.com.

pest control alternatives in crop production becomes imperative. Consequently, there has been an increased research attention on the use of natural compounds as a poisoning option to replace agro-chemicals. These natural compounds also known as botanical insecticides which the Neem seed oil is one of them constitute desirable alternatives to the synthetic pesticides. They are best suited for use in organic food production in industrialized countries. Nevertheless, they can still play a much greater role in the developing countries as a new class of eco-friendly products for pest control. These botanical pesticides should be incorporated in the pest management programs. When, this is done, they can serve as alternatives to synthetic pesticides, or used in combination them, or more so in rotation with other pesticides. The application of the above options could delay the development of control resistance in pests. The plant based insecticides induce acute toxicity to pests which deters them from causing great economic losses at the pre- and post- harvest stages of crop production. The Neem amongst other plant species is the most researched and commercially exploited in pest management. The substances with pesticidal properties are found in all parts of the Neem tree, however, the greatest concentration of it is found in the seed. The Neem seed contains an active ingredient called the Azadirachtin which consists of more than 25 different but closely related compounds. It is extracted from the seed kernel in the form of oil, cake or powder. This Neem Seed Kernel Extracts (NSKE) viz-a-viz the Neem Seed Oil (NO) and the Neem Cake (NC) are used in various fields and horticultural crops for pest management. The Azadirachtin was reported to be active against over 550 insect species. The NO is a powerful and natural insecticide capable of disrupting the life cycle of insects at all stages. Its efficacy and availability makes it a great resource for the poor farmers. The modes of action of NSKE on insect pests include direct effect on insect reproduction which is manifested in their growth reduction, increased mortality rate, abnormal and delayed moults. This research explains the production, uses and benefits of the Neem seed oil.

Keywords: Neem seed oil, pests, Azadirachtin, production, uses

INTRODUCTION: SOURCE OF THE NEEM SEED OIL

The Neem oil is a botanical insecticide derived from the tree *Azadirachta indica* (A. Juss), and is valued for centuries worldwide as an important source of phytochemicals for use in human health and pest control. The Neem tree (*Azadirachta indica* A. Juss) is a member of the Meliaceae family that originates from the India subcontinent. It can tolerate high temperatures as well as poor or degraded soil. The young leaves are reddish to purple in colour, while the mature leaves are bright green, consisting of petiole, lamina, and the base that attaches the leaf to the stem. It may bear two small lateral leaf-like structures known as stipules (Norten and Pütz, 1999). The Neem tree is widely distributed throughout tropical Africa in both dry and humid areas for shade, for reforestation programmes and in plantations for the production of compounds which have toxic, antifeedant and repellent properties against insects (FAO 1988). The tree is widely distributed extensively in Nigeria and many parts of the West African countries such as Sierra Leone, Ghana, Sudan, Ethiopia and the other parts of the Eastern and Southern Africa. It is used for pest control in crude aqueous formulation (Dialoke et al. 2015a).

The Neem oil contains at least 100 biologically active compounds. Amongst the major constituents are triterpenes known as limonoids, and the Azadirachtin (Figure 1a), which appears to cause 90% of the effect on most pests. The active ingredient Azadirachtin was isolated from the seeds of *A. indica* by David Morgan (Butterworth and Morgan 1968) and its full structural determination was completed some 17 years later concurrently in the laboratories of Steven Ley, W Kraus and K Nakanishi (Bilton et al. 1987, Kraus et al. 1987, Turner et al. 1987). The Azadirachtin, a complex tetranortri-terpenoid limonoid from the Neem seeds is the main component responsible for both antifeedant and toxic effects in insects. Other limonoid and sulphur-containing compound with repellent, antiseptic, contraceptive, antipyretic and antiparasitic properties are found elsewhere in the tree, e.g., the leaves, the flowers, the bark, and the roots (Mordue (Luntz) and Nisbet, (2000). The antifeedant effects of Neem were the first to be described scientifically. In 1952, Heinrich Schmutterer recorded desert locusts (*Schistocerca gregaria* (Forskal) that refused to feed on Neem. (Mordue (Luntz) and Nisbet, (2000).

The compound has a melting point of 160°C and molecular weight of 720 g/mol. Other most common active components present in the Neem tree include meliantriol, nimbin, nimbidin, nimbinin, nimbolides, fatty acids (oleic, stearic, and palmitic), and salannin (Figure 1b). The main Neem product is the oil extracted from the seeds by different techniques. The other parts of the Neem tree contain less Azadirachtin, but are also used for oil extraction (Nicoletti, et al. 2012). It has been suggested that the content of Azadirachtin in the seeds can be increased by artificial infection with arbuscular mycorrhiza (Venkateswarlu et al. 2008). The Neem seed oil contains the major concentrations of these active compounds along with many fatty acids like oleic acids, stearic acid, palmitic acid, linoleic acid etc. Lesser amounts of these active compounds are also found in the Neem leaves and bark.

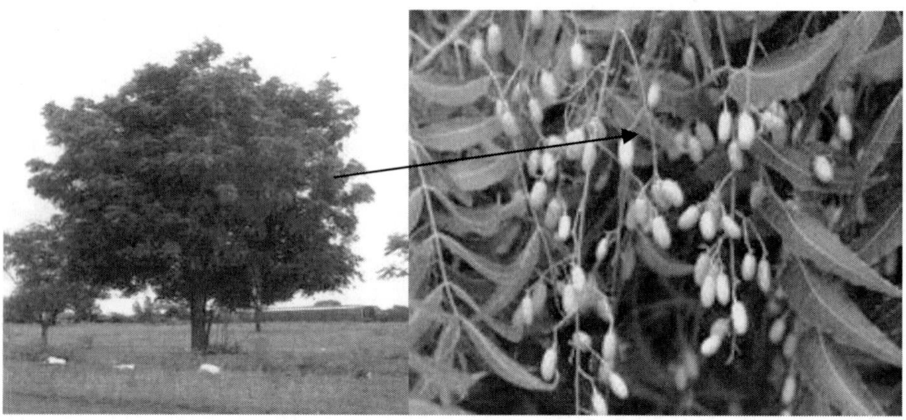

Plate 1. Matured neem tree produced ripe neem fruits (arrowed).

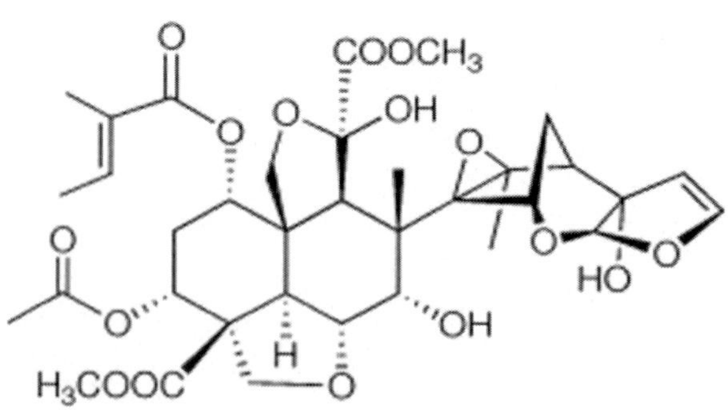

Figure 1.a. Chemical Structure of Azadirachtin, the Main Component of the Neem Oil. (Adopted from Estefania, et al. (2016).

Neem Active Compounds	Functions
Azadirachtin	It provides repellent, anti-hormonal and anti-feedant properties
Nimbin	It provides anti-inflammatory, anti-pyretic, anti-histamine and anti-fungal properties
Nimbidin	It provides anti-bacterial, anti-ulcer, analgesic, anti-arhythmical and anti-fungal properties
Nimbidol	provides anti-tubercular, anti-protozoa and anti-pyretic properties
Sodium nimbinate	It provides diuretic, spermicidal and anti-arthritic properties
Gedunin	It provides vasodilator, anti-malaria anti-fungal properties
Salannin	It provides repellent properties
Quercetin	It provides anti-protozoal, anti-oxidant and anti-inflammatory and anti-bacterial properties.

Figure 1.b. Functions of the Active Compounds in the Neem Tree (Adopted from www.neemfoundation.org.).

MECHANISMS OF ACTION

The Azadirachtin can act as a feeding deterrent or as an "antifeedant" to insects that feed on leaves and other plant parts. The oil is considered a contact insecticide, presenting systemic and translaminar activity (Cox, 2002).It has a broad spectrum of action, inhibiting feeding, affecting hormone function in juveniles reducing ecdysone, deregulating growth, altering development and reproduction, suppressing fertility, sterilizing, repelling oviposition, and disrupting molting processes so that the immature larvae cannot develop into adults (Schmutterer, 1990; Brahmachari, 2004). After treatment with neem-based pesticides, you may see insects with crippled, distorted wing or the immature larvae and nymphs remaining in an immature stage before they then die. Some soft-skinned insect larvae may be killed by direct contact with the spray. The adults are not killed by the growth regulating properties of Azadirachtin but their mating and sexual communication may be disrupted which results in reduced fecundity. The Neem oil works in a number of different ways. The oil forms a coating on the insect's body, blocking the breathing openings and suffocating the insect. It also has a repellent effect on certain insects and mites.

Due to its insect growth regulating properties, it is most effective against the immature stages of insects. For example, the immature larvae of many species in the lepidoptera family (moths and butterflies) are particularly sensitive to azadirachtin (Schmutterer, 1990). The Neem products may be registered for use on certain fruits, herbs and vegetables in addition to ornamentals. For edible crops, some neem-based products may be used up to the day of harvest (Quarles, 1994). The effects of combination of botanical compounds vary in their mechanisms of action. Little is known about the mode of action of azadirachtin as a feeding inhibitor, although it is possible that it stimulates cells involved in feeding inhibition, causing weakness and pest death (Brahmachari, 2004).

The Azadirachtin, salannin, and other limonoids present in the Neem Oil inhibit ecdysone 20-monooxygenase, the enzyme responsible for catalyzing the final step in conversion of ecdysone to the active hormone, 20-hydroxyecdysone, which controls the insect metamorphosis process. However, these effects are probably secondary to the action of azadirachtin in blocking microtubule formation in actively dividing cells (Morgan, 2009). Moreover, the Azadirachtin can inhibit the release of prothoracicotropic hormone and allatotropins from the brain-corpus cardiacum complex, resulting in problems of fertility and fecundity (Mulla and Su, 1999). Meliantriol and salannin also act to inhibit the feeding of insects, (Wilps et al. 1992). This Azadirachtin components can also interfere in mitosis, in the same way as colchicine, and has direct histopathological effects on insect gut epithelial cells, muscles, and fatty tissues, resulting in restricted movement and decreased flight activity (Wilps et al. 1992; Qias et al. 2014).

BENEFITS OF THE NEEM PRODUCTS TO MANKIND

Environmental Safety

The major factors that have stimulated the use of neem-based products for pest control in agriculture are ecological and toxicological factors (low toxicity to non-target organisms), as well as economic factors. A little quantity of the product can provide effective pest control, (Ogbuewu, et al. 2011). The Neem products do not persist in the environment and can be degraded by ultraviolet light and rainfall. Many neem-products have low mammalian toxicity. They also act as natural fungicides that control diseases caused by pathogenic organisms such as fungi, and bacteria. Because many neem products degrade quickly, they may have reduced effect on non-target beneficial organisms compared to some of the more traditional pesticides. Some researchers have discovered few effects on many insect predators such as spiders, earwigs, and ants but flower fly larvae are very sensitive to neem sprays.

IPM Compatibility

The Neem-based materials are compatible with integrated pest management (IPM) (Schmutterer, 1990). Regular scouting helps to insure the early detection of immature stages of many insects. Azadirachtin is compatible with insecticidal soap, superior horticultural oil and *Bacillus thuringiensis* (Bt) (Locke, 1994). The application of the Neem oil prevents the germination and penetration of some fungal spores (Locke, 1994). In one study, researchers discovered that a one percent Neem oil treatment was effective in managing powdery mildew on hydrangeas, lilacs and phlox (Locke, 1994). As earlier mentioned, the azadirachtin has a number of different modes of action. It is less likely that insects or pathogens will develop resistance to Neem products compared to materials with a single mode of action.

Table 1. An Overview of Repellent Neem Oil Efficacy from Literature review

Plant	Location	Other Names	Repellent compound(s)	Tested mode of use	Repellency % protection	Study type	Ref.
MELIACEAE	India Srilanka			direct burning (leaves)	70% protection from mosquitoes from 2 hours	field study in Guinea Bissau	Ansari, et al. 2005
	China Brazil			Periodic thermal expulsion (leaves)	24.5% from An.protection gambiae spp	semi-field study in Kenya	Dremova et al. (1971).
	Bolivia Pakistan Ethiopia	Neem	Azadirachtin Saponins	1% Neem oil volatilized in a kerosene lamp	94.2% protection from Anopheles spp 80% protection from Culex spp.	field study in India	Kwon et al. (2010).
Azadirachta Indica	Guinea Bissau						
	Kenya Tanzania			2% Neem oil applied topically	56.75% protection from mosquitoes for 4 hours	field study in Bolivia	Sakuku, et al. 2008

Adopted from PMC (2011).

Medicinal

The Neem seed oil is highly advantageous over broad-spectrum conventional pesticides. It affects only target pest and closely related organisms. It requires only a small quantity to be productive. It decomposes quickly. Among the botanical insecticides currently marketed, the Neem oil is one of the least toxic to humans but very lethal in the control of many pests (Rehman et al. 2014). It is known to be an excellent mosquito repellent, especially the *Anopheles stephensi* and *A. culicifacies* group, (Table 1) Lucantoni et al.2006; Rehman et al. 2014). A formulated Neem oil repellent DEET when rubbed as pomade repels mosquitoes (Syed and Leal, 2008). You can mix it with coconut oil and apply it over your body as well for protection against mosquitoes. It is believed that in India, small children are fed with Neem oil as a type of cure-all. Several field studies from India have shown very high efficacy of Neem-based preparations (Singh, et al. 1996; Sharmaetal. 1993; Caraballo, 2000). This is contrasting with findings of intermediate repellency by other researchers (Barnard and Xue, 2004; Moore, et al. 2002).However, these contrasting results could differ from each other due Methodologies, and the solvents used to prepare the repellents. For many years now in Nigeria and India, a Neem twig is what people used as a make-do toothbrush. It fights germs, maintains the alkaline levels in saliva, keeps bacteria at bay, treats swollen gums and also gives you whiter teeth.

Limitations of the Neem Oil

The greatest limitation of Neem oil is its low stability under field conditions, due to mainly a high rate of photodegradation of its active ingredients, as it also has residual time and slow killing rates compared to other conventional pesticides (Isman, 2006, Miresmailli and Isman, 2014; de Oliveira et al. 2014). These uncertainties hinder the large scale use of Neem oil. It has been observed through several studies on Neem oil that due to its low residual power, multiple applications are required in order to control pests, which can increase selection pressure on the pest population, possibly leading to their resistance (Ghosh, et al. 2012; Tangtrakulwanich and Reddy 2014; Siegwart et al. 2015). The Neem oil contains a group of active ingredients with different chemical characteristics which was believed to make the development of insect resistance virtually impossible. But currently most of the studies on the Neem oil revealed that its effectiveness against many pests has to do with its feeding deterrent action, so their indiscriminate use could result in the development of resistance (Tangtrakulwanich and Reddy 2014; Mpumi et al. 2016). Feng and Isman (1995) evaluated the behavior of two lines of *Myzus persicae*, which were exposed to pure Azadirachtin or to refined Neem seed extract at the same concentration as Azadirachtin. It was found that after forty generations, the line treated with Azadirachtin had developed ninefold greater resistance to azadirachtin, compared to a control line, whereas the line treated with the extract did not show resistance. Because the Neem oil is an insect growth regulator, it is only effective against the immature stages of insects. Rescue treatments will not be effective. You will not see an immediate knockdown effect and insects may continue to feed. However, due to its repellent effects, the rate of insect feeding will be reduced. The chemical compositions of Neem oil are mainly determined by the genetic factors inherent in the Neem tree. Also environmental factors and the type of extraction method can lead to significant differences in composition. As a result, there is no standard active ingredient in the composition of this Neem oil, which limits its application in the control of agricultural pests (Ghosh et al. 2012; Tangtrakulwanich and Reddy 2014; Siegwart et al. 2015). Phytotoxicity (damage to plants) may be of concern for certain formulations of the Neem -based products with flowers being particularly sensitive. Newly transplanted plants with limited root development or plants that are wilted or under stress should not be treated (Stone, 1992). Neem products are mainly used by developing countries in a crude formulation form because of lack of facilities to refine the products. However, one of the main problems facing the commercial development of neem is a lack of industrial interest, largely due to the difficulty of patenting natural products, as well as a shortage of scientific evidence to support claims regarding the benefits of these substances and as a result the products are not widely publicized in the farming community or elsewhere (Pant et al. 2016). These uncertainties and all other impediments must have to be resolved so that a full potential use of the Neem oil for human use and pests control can be exploited.

PROCESSING /PRODUCTION

Aqueous Production of Neem Insecticides

The production of azadirachtin is carried out from the kernels of the Neem seeds (*Azadrachta indica*). Collect only good quantity of ripe neem fruits which are yellow not green from a mature tree of 9-17 years old. These odoriferous azadirachtin which contains biologically active secondary metabolites such as alkaloids, phenolics, and terpenoids are extracted from the Neem seeds, using extraction methods employing aqueous or organic solvents, or steam distillation. De-pulp the harvested seeds by removing the outer layer. After this, spread the seeds in an open breezy place in the shade of a tree or house with mats to dry for a few days. Do not expose the seeds to rain or direct sunshine. This is very important as the active ingredient in the seed called Azadirachtin loses its efficacy when it is exposed to light heat and sunlight. Bear in mind that the seeds must be well dried before storing them to avoid the growth of moulds which will eventually spoil the seeds. Store the seeds in well aerated baskets or jute gunny sacks. Do not put them in plastic bags. This will keep moisture inside and make the seeds rot. The shelf life can be one year from the date of manufacturing if kept under normal condition.

Remove the seed coat. For this, you need a large mortar which you do not use for grinding other food products. This is because Neem is very bitter and will give an unpleasant flavor to anything you grind in the mortar. Place 0.5-0.8kg of the seeds in the mortar and pound them very gently not hard but enough to break off the seed coat exposing the kernel inside. Next separate the broken seed coats from the kernel by winnowing them in a light wind. Then put a handful of clean kernels into the mortar and this time pound vigorously until you produce a fine powder. Diagram in Figure 2, explains to the local farmers the technology involved in making aqueous solution of Neem products for use in the farm. It will be advisable for the farmer to make as much powder as he may use in few weeks, because the insect repelling properties does not last long once it is made into a powdered form, especially if it is exposed to light or heat. Apart from crude production of the Neem extract, the Neem oil can also be formulated to increase its efficacy, its storability and also to decrease the potential phytotoxicity. The Neem oil is less systemic because it is insoluble in water. It should be formulated to make it systemic, so as to enhance its efficacy on sucking pests. To overcome these hurdles, better formulations are being developed (Senguttuvan, 2001).

Scientific Production of Oil from Different Parts of the Neem Plant

Harvest and weigh 900g of ripe Neem seeds, 900g of unripe Neem seeds, and 150g kg of Neem leaves (Dialoke et al. 2015a). Air dry and oven dry at 60°C for 12 hours in other to stabilize the moisture content and there after crush them with different mortar and pestle and put in different containers. Weigh with a sensitive weighing balance, 100g of the crushed ripe and unripe Neem seed respectively and 150 g of the crushed leave, (Dialoke et al. 2015a). Put them in two separate litres specimen bottles containing petroleum spirit and shake for two hours with a reciprocating shaker. Afterwards, put the mixture in a thimble instrument and extract oil with the use of thermal soxlet apparatus. It is very important to air dry the extracted oil so that the traces of the solvent can evaporate. The extracted oil from different Neem plant parts are stored in a refrigerator under 4-10°C using plastics with tight cover and subsequently used for research trial on okra pests. The result of this is presented in Table 2 (Dialoke et al. 2015a).

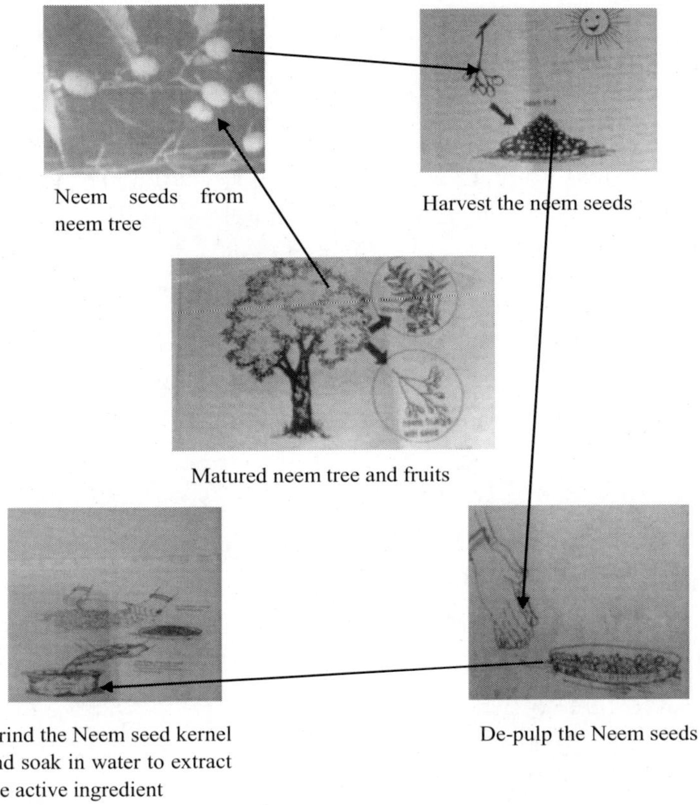
Neem seeds from neem tree
Harvest the neem seeds
Matured neem tree and fruits
Grind the Neem seed kernel and soak in water to extract the active ingredient
De-pulp the Neem seeds

Figure 2. Preparation of insecticide from the Neem tree (Adopted from Emosairue, 2007).

NEEM APPLICATION IN MEDICINE AND AGRICULTURE

For thousands of years, the Indian farmers have been aware of the insecticidal properties of the Neem tree. Its branches were hung in granaries to protect stored grain from insect attack. The Neem extract has been used for centuries in folk medicine for the treatment of conditions such as malaria, ulcers, cardiovascular disease, and skin problems (Figure 3) (Estefania, et al. 2016). Despite the limited existence of clinical trials to support these therapeutic claims, the use of Neem has grown over time, and it is an important component of Ayurvedic medicine (medical knowledge) developed in India about 7,000 years ago; (Girish and Shankara Bhat, 2008; Ogbuewu, et al. 2011).

Since the 1970s, the scientists in Europe and the United States of America became interested in Neem because of its insecticidal properties plus its low toxicity to mammals (Schmutterer, 1990). The Neem seed oil has been used in Agriculture to control some major insect pests in the farmers' field and storage chamber some centuries of years ago. Research studies were conducted at the Department of Crop Science and Technology, Teaching and Research Farm at Federal University of Technology, Owerri, Nigeria (plate 2) on the pests of some specific crops. Owerri, is located in the rain forest belt, longitude 7° 12′ E and latitude 5° 27′ N of equator in Imo State Nigeria. Different rates of Neem seed oil and oil from different parts of Neem tree were used to control the pests of soybean and okra. Also formulated neem seed oil at different rates and frequencies were used to monitor different pests on pigeonpea plants. The treatments comprised three rates of formulated Neem seed oil (2 ml (4.2 ℓ in 840 litres of water ha^{-1}), 4 ml (8.3 ℓ in 840 litres of waterha^{-1}), 6 ml (12.5 ℓ in 840 litres of water ha^{-1}), untreated plot (0 ℓ ha^{-1}) and synthetic pyrethroid (Cyperforce (cypermethrin 30g/l +dimethoate 250 g/l EC) at 0.72 ml (1.5 ℓ in 840 litres of water ha^{-1}) as checks) while spraying regime were, three (3) intervals of application (once in a week, once in two weeks, and once in three weeks).. At spraying time, each rate was mixed with one litre of clean water.

The actions of Neem seed oil which have been described in specific groups of insects in Nigeria include actions against (i) several soybean pests (plates 4-12)(ii) Coleoptera: pigeonpea leaf beetle, *Aulacophora vinula* (Dialoke et al. 2015b), okra flea beetle, *Podagrica* spp (plates 15 a-c) (Dialoke et al. 2015a), (iii) Hemiptera: podsucking bugs, e.g., *Riptortus dentipes* (Dialoke et al. 2014b), (iv) Thymnsoptera: e.g., Thrips; Dialoke et al.2014c; (v) Lepidoptera: podborer e.g., *Helicoverpa armigera* (Dialoke et al. 2017). In other countries, several studies on antifeeding effect and increased larvae mortality (Mancebo et al. 2002; Michereff-ilho et al. 2008; Tavares et al. 2010), of the Neem seed oil have equally been carried out on the following pests (i) Lepidoptera: e.g., *Helicoverpa armigera*

(Ahmad et al. 2015), Bollworms, Armyworms, Fruitworms, Caterpillers, Leaf folder, Leaf miners, Borers (Pod borer, Fruit borer), Leaf hopper, Diamond backmoth,Cutworms, etc. (ii) Hemiptera: podsucking bugs, e.g.,*Riptortus dentipes*, etc., early death of nymphs is due to inhibition of development and ecdysis defects (Weathersbee and Mckenzie, 2005; Senthil Nathan et al. 2006; Formentini et al. 2016) Insect vectors e.g., Aphids, Whitefly, Mealy bugs, Thrips, *Mamestra brassicae* (Seljasen and Meadow,2006), (iii) Coleoptera: *Nilaparvata lugens Stal* Senthil Nathan et al. 2006;*Pieris brassicae* (Hasan and Shafig Ansari, 2011), and *Spodoptera frugiperda* (Tavares et al. 2010), (iv) Neuroptera: severe damage in the midgut cells of larvae, injury and cell death during the replacement of midgut epithelium, and changes in cocoons, with increased porosity and decreased wall thickness affecting pupation (Scudeler et al. 2013,2014, Scudeler and dos Santos, 2013).

Arachnid targets include *Hyalomma anatolicum excavatum* (Abdel-Shafy and Zayed, 2002) and *Sarcoptes scabie* var. cuniculi larvae (Xu et al. 2010). In another class, the Arachnida, exposure of the Ixodidae group to the Neem oil decreased egg hatching and caused malformation, deformities, and death of larvae and adults (Abdel-Shafy and Zayed, 2002).Target crops in which the actions of neem seed oil on insect pests have been demonstrated are as follows, soybean, cotton, rice, pigeonpea, tea, chickpea, sunflower, okra, cauliflower, tobacco, cabbage, tomato and lots more.

Contribution of Neem Products to Organic Agriculture

The eco-friendly qualities of the Neem support its contribution to organic agricultural production systems that are more sustainable and do not generate chemical residues (plants and crops are grown without the use of any agrochemicals). The use of Neem also helps to maintain soil productivity, ensuring longer production times. In quest for organic food production all over the world, organic agriculture can be a viable alternative production method for farmers, even though there are many challenges that have to be overcome. The interesting thing is to appreciate the role of Neem products which is that it can effectively contribute to organic agriculture, being used as organic pesticides and as soil fertilizers. In addition, growing concerns about conventional agriculture and the demand for products that do not generate waste justify increased adoption of the use of biopesticides by farmers, which contributes to the growth of organic agriculture (Dubey, et al.2010; Seufert, et al.2012; Gahukar, 2014).

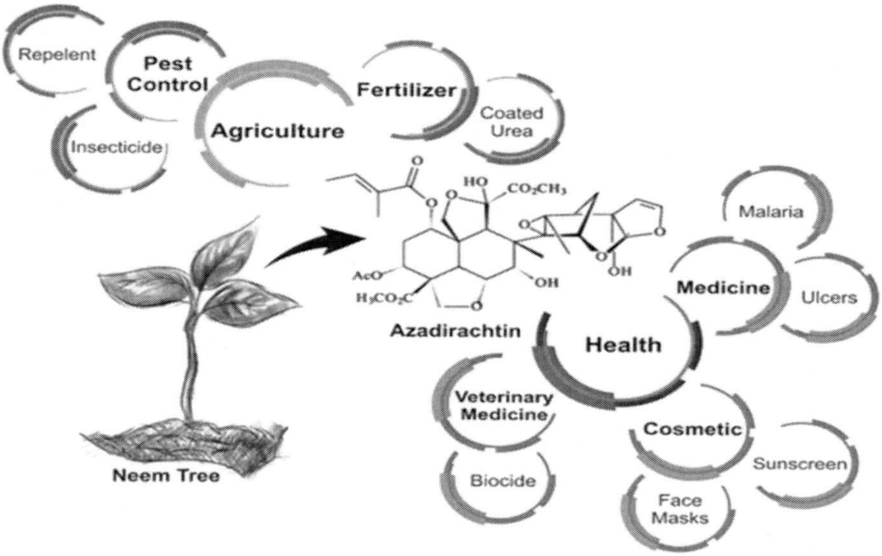

Figure 3. Potential applications of azadirachtin in different areas (Adopted from Estefania, et al. 2016).

Indian farmers have traditionally used de-oiled Neem cake as a fertilizer in their fields. The dual activity of neem cake as fertilizer and pest repellent has made it a favoured input. Neem leaves have also been used to enrich the soil. Together, they are widely used in Nigeria and India to fertilize cash crops. When Neem cake is ploughed into the soil it also protects plant roots from nematodes and white ants. Farmers in Southern parts of India puddle Neem leaves into flooded rice fields before the rice seedlings are transplanted.

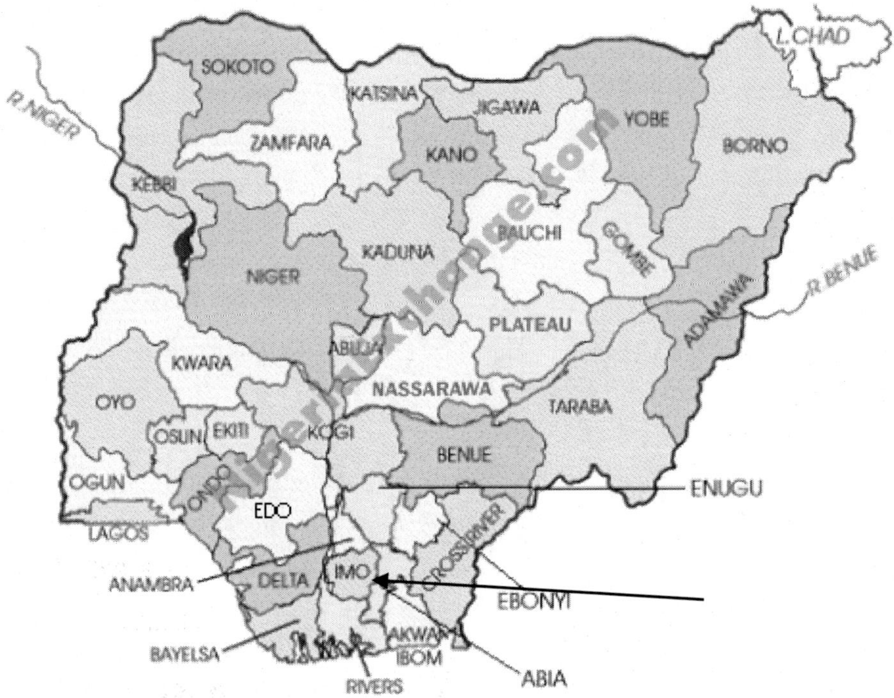

Plate 2. Map of Nigeria showing location of Imo State (arrowed).

Application of the Neem seed cake to crops provides them with various nutrients. Besides, the Neem seed cake also reduces the number of soil insect pests, fungi, bacteria and nematodes and protects the crop from damage caused by these organisms (Akhtar, 2000). The Neem seed cake can also reduce alkalinity in the soil by producing organic acids when mixed with the soil. For plant development, the neem seed cake is also an excellent fertilizer and releases 56.6% nitrogen at 60 days (Koul; Isman; Ketkar, 1990). It has also been reported to serve as a protective effect against nematodes, due to toxic substances released through volatilization, exudation, leaching and decomposition (Akhtar, 2000), then reducing nematodes population (Khan; Alam; Ahmad, 1974). In tobacco, which was incorporated Neem cake, there was an increase in the production, even on infected soil with *M. incognita* (Desai et al. 1979) Various concentrations of the neem over the development of earthworm, which is essential for soil fertility (Mayilswami; Reid, 2010), caused no negative effect at high concentration and a slight increase in the development of the worms. Although the Neem in commercially recommended concentration of extract, does not harm earthworms (*Pheretima peguana*), but a high concentrations of Neem is cytotoxic to them (Muangphra; Gooneratne, 2011).

COMMERCIAL PRODUCTS DERIVED FROM NEEM (*AZADIRACHTA INDICA*)

The Neem has acquired commercial recognition due to its various beneficial properties, which have been extensively investigated over time. Compared to conventional chemicals, which are generally persistent in the environment and highly toxic, botanical pesticides are biodegradable and leave no harmful residues. Most botanical pesticides are non-phytotoxic and are also more selective toward the target pest. In terms of commercial applications, the neem as a biopesticides can provide substantial economic advantages, since the infrastructure required is inexpensive, compared to conventional pesticides (Pant, et al. 2016). Several patents related to processes and products based on neem have been deposited in the United States, India, Japan, Australia, and elsewhere. Table 2, shows some of the main commercial products based on the Neem which are currently in use all over the world. Many of the products derived from Neem are manufactured by crushing the seeds and other plant parts, followed by the use of solvents to extract the active ingredients possessing pesticide ingredients. The different methods and techniques employed to obtain the Neem products can result in different concentrations of the active compounds, as well as different biological effectiveness (Roychoudhury, 2016).

Table 2. Neem Applications and Commercial Products Available Worldwide

Application	Products	Manufacturer
Fertilizer	Ozoneem Cake®	Ozone Biotech (India)
	Plan "B" Organics – Neem Cake®	Plan "B" Organics (USA)
	Fortuneem Cake®	Fortune Biotech (USA)
	Bio Neem Oil Foliar®	FUSA – Fertilizers of the USA
	Neem Cake®	Unibell Corporation (Russia)
	Ozoneem Coat®	Ozone Biotech (India)
	Parker Neem Coat®	Parker Neem (India)
	Neem Urea Guard®	Neemex (India)
	Fortuneem Coat®	Fortune Biotech (USA)
	Azadirachtin-based products	
Agrochemical	AZA-Direct®	Gowan Company (USA)
	Neemix 4.5®	Certis (USA)
	Fortune Aza 3% EC®	Fortune Biotech (USA)
	Azamax®	UPL Ltda. (Brazil)
	Neemazal Technical®	E.I.D. Parry Ltd. (India)
	Ecosense®	Agro Logistic Systems Inc. (USA)
	Safer Brand 3 in 1	Woodstream Corp. (Canada)
	Garden Spray®	
	Azatin XL®	OHP Inc. (USA)
	Azact CE®	EPP Ltda. (Brazil)
	Neem oil	
	Triact 70 EC®	Certis Company (USA)
	BioNeem®	Woodstream Corporation (USA)
	Shubhdeep Neem Oil®	King Agro Food (India)
	DalNeem®	Dalquim Ltda. (Brazil)
	OzoNeem Oil®	Ozone Biotech (India)
	NeemDrop®	Neem India Products Ltd. (India)

Adopted from Estefania, et al. (2016).

RESEARCH INFORMATION ON CONSEQUENCES OF FEEDING INSECTS WITH THE NEEM OIL

Insects belonging to different orders differ in their behavior responses to this active ingredient of Neem, the Azadirachtin (Table 3).The order Lepidoptera are extremely sensitive to the Azadirachtin and show effective antifeedancies from <1-50 ppm, depending upon species (Mordue (Luntz) and Nisbet, 2000). Coleoptera, Hemiptera and Homoptera are less sensitive to Azadirachtin behaviorally with up to 100% antifeedancy being achieved at 100-600 ppm.Though there are some aphid species which also show behavioral sensitivity e.g., strawberry aphid, (Mordue and Nisbet, 2000). The Orthoptera show an enormous range in sensitivity from *S. gregaria* (a polyphagous species which has chemoreceptors finely tuned to many plant secondary compounds) to *Locusta migratoria* (L.) (a graminaceous species which does not have chemoreceptors tunes to feeding deterrents) to the extreme insensitivity of *Melanoplus sanguinipes* (Fab.), the North American Plains grasshopper which is an evolutionary sense has never encountered *A. indica* and has no chemoreceptors responding to Azadirachtin (Mordue (Luntz) and Nisbet, 2000). Such 'primary' (or gustatory) antifeedancy - 'the inability to ingest resulting from the perception of the antifeedant at a sensory level' (Schmutterer, 1985), is responsible for crop protection in several species of Lepidoptera and Desert locusts (*S. gregaria*) are very sensitive to azadirachtin and fail to feed on sugar impregnated discs when the compound is present at concentrations of 0.01 ppm and above (Mordue (Luntz) et al. 1996). The Azadirachtin sprayed onto barley seedlings infested with *S. gregaria* nymphs protect plants at low doses (2 ppm) (Nasiruddin and Mordue (Luntz) 1993). *Spodoptera littoralis* (African cotton leafworm), *Spodoptera frugiperda*; (fall armyworm), *Heliothis virescens* (F.) (tobacco budworm) and *Helicoverpa armigera* (Hüb.) (old world bollworm) also respond behaviorally to low concentrations of azadirachtin and are prevented from feeding on discs impregnated with the compound at concentrations of 0.1 - 10 ppm dependent upon species (Blaney et al. 1990, Simmonds et al. 1990, Mordue (Luntz) et al. 1998). The comparison of the antifeedant and toxic properties of azadirachtin with various less structurally complex putative biosynthetic precursors against larvae of *Spodoptera littoralis* (Boisd.), *S. gregaria* and *Oncopeltus fasciatus* Dallas (milkweed bug) has shown that toxicity to insects (severe growth and moult disruption) was only observed with azadirachtin.

Table 3. Behavioural Sensitivity of Insects to Azadirachtin: The Effective Dose (ED50) which causes 50% of Feeding

	ED_{50} (ppm)
Lepidopteara	<0.001-50
Coleoptera	100-500
Hemiptera	100-500
Hymenoptera	100-500
Orthoptera	0.001->1000

Adopted from Mordue (Luntz) and Nisbet, (2000).

In addition, for the Azadirachtin itself, whereas the toxic insect growth regulatory (IGR) effects are seen in all species, antifeedancy varies markedly between Insect Order and species within orders (Mordue (Luntz) and Blackwell 1993). The antifeedant effects observed in these species are highly correlated with the sensory response of chemoreceptors on the insect mouthparts (Mordue (Luntz) et al. 1998). Feeding behavior depend upon both neural input from the insects' chemical senses (taste receptor on tarsi, mouthparts and oral cavity) and central nervous integration of this 'sensory code'. The Azadirachtin stimulates specific 'deterrent' cells in chemoreceptors and also blocks the firing of 'sugar' receptor cells which normally stimulate feeding (Blaney et al. 1990, Simmonds et al. 1990, Mordue (Luntz) et al. 1999). This results in starvation and death of these species by feeding deterrency alone.

However, in most other species of phytophagous insect, crop protection results from a combination of antifeedancy and physiological effects due to the ingestion of azadirachtin. These physiological effects include 'secondary' antifeedancy whereby feeding is reduced post-ingestively. These "secondary" antifeedant effects include 'a reduction in food consumption and digestive efficiency subsequent to, and as a consequence of, ingestion, application or injection of the antifeedant' (Schmutterer, 1985).

The secondary antifeedant effects result from the disturbance of hormonal and/or other physiological system e.g., movement of food through the gut, inhibitions of digestive enzyme production, effects on the stomatogastric nervous system etc. (Mordue (Luntz) et al. 1985, Koul and

Isman 1991, Timmins and Reynolds 1992, Trumm and Dorn 2000). For example, some locusts injected with azadirachtin, which by-passes the taste receptors, showed a reduced ingestion of food as seen by faecal pellet production (Nasiruddin and Mordue (luntz) 1993). Hemipteran insects feeding on tobacco seedlings which had been systemically treated with 500 ppm azadirachtin were shown initially to feed normally but, after termination of the initial feed, the interval prior to the next subsequent feed was significantly increased and feeding activity thereafter was suppressed (Nisbet et al. 1993). Also aphids which had fed on artificial diets containing much lower concentration of azadirachtin (25 ppm) exhibited no signs of primary antifeedant effects during an initial 24h period of access to the diets but their feeding rate fell drastically in the subsequent 24h period (Nisbet et al. 1994).

A consequence of interrupted feeding activity can be an effect on the ability of insects to transmit pathogens. Aphids require extended feeding periods to acquire persistently-transmitted luteoviruses (e.g., potato leafroll virus, PLRV) from plants. Treatment of PLRV-infected tobacco plants with azadirachtin reduced sustained feeding by *Myzus persicae* (Sulzer) (peach-potato aphid) and reduced the ability of aphids to acquire and transmit PLRV. However, azadirachtin does not always reduce the spread of plant virus diseases by aphids. Treatment of uninfected seedlings with the same concentrations of azadirachtin (500 ppm) failed to prevent them from becoming infected when viruliferous aphids fed on them (Nisbet et al. 1996a). The successful infection of a plant with luteoviruses is dependent upon the transfer of aphid saliva to the plant, a process which may be brief by comparison with the time required for virus acquisition by the aphid, and is not overcome by the presence of the antifeedant. Similarly, the azadirachtin failed to protect seedlings from infections with a non-persistently transmitted potyvirus (potato virus y) from viruliferous aphids (Nisbet 1992).

EFFECTS OF THE AZADIRACHTIN ON THE PHYSIOLOGY OF INSECT PESTS

The Azadirachtin effects on the physiology of insect pests are much more consistent than the antifeedant effects. It results from interference with growth and moulting, interference with reproduction and interference with cellular processes (Table 4, Mordue (Luntz) and Nisbet, (2000). In all species tested, the dose response effects can be seen in reduced growth, increased mortalities, abnormal moults and delayed moults. These effects are related to disruption of endocrine system controlling growth and moulting. The moulting effects are due to a disruption in the synthesis and release of ecdysteroids (moulting hormone) and other classes of hormones and this can be demonstrated by accurately timed injections of azadirachtin into the haemoulymph of 5th instar nymphs of *L. migratoria* (Mordue (Luntz)et al.1986). Measurements of haemolymph ecdysteroid levels by radioimmuno assay (RAY) revealed the normal peak of hormone release at day 8 of an 11-day instar. In those insects injected with azadirachtin before hormone release, ecdysteroid release is blocked entirely and the insects die before the moult after an extended instar. For those injected at the start of ecdysone release, the peak is delayed and its decline slow down Mordue (Luntz) and Nisbet, (2000).This prevents the release of eclosion hormone which controls the motor programme of eclosion or moulting and these insects also die before they moult. Finally, if injected at the peak of ecdysone release, the moult initiation proceeds but the insects die during ecdyses unable to swallow enough air to extricate themselves from the old cuticle (plate 3 a-c).

Azadirachtin prevents the proliferation of Sf9 cells *in vitro* and alters both the protein content and abundance in those cells (Figure 4). Rembold and Annadurai 1993). It therefore appears from these observations that azadirachtin operates at the cellular level by disrupting protein synthesis and secretion events. At the molecular level by altering or preventing the transcription of proteins expressed during and/or translation of proteins expressed during periods of rapid protein synthesis e.g., in piding cells or cells forming new assemblages of organelles or cytoskeleton (Mordue (Luntz) and Nisbet, (2000).

Table 4. The Overall Effects of the Azadirachtin against Insects

Effects	Target	Mode of action
Primary	mouthpart and other	Deterrent cell stimulation
Antifidancy	chemoreceptors	sugar cell inhibition
Secondary	Gut	Peristalsis inhibited
Antifidancy		Enzyme production reduced
Insect growth Regulation	Cuticle	Alterations to ecdysteroid and JH titres by blockage and release of morphogenic peptides leading to moulting defects
Sterility	Reproductive organs	Alterations to ecdysteroid and JH titres leading to reduction in number of viable eggs and life progeny
Cellular processes	Dividing cells	Blockage of cell division post metaphase in meiosis and mitosis
	Muscles	Loss of muscle tone
	Cell synthetic Machinery	Blockage of digestive enzyme production in gut. Inhibition of protein synthesis in various tissues.

Adopted from Mordue (Luntz) and Nisbet, (2000).

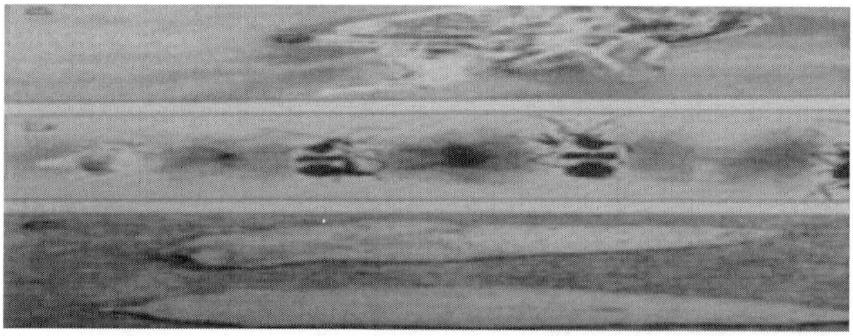

(a)

(b)

(c)

Plate 3-a-c. Moulting abnormalities caused by azadirachtin treatment, a-desert locust (*S.gragaria*) showing death at ecdysis (× 1.5); b-milkweed bug (*O. fasciatus*) showing moulting defects (× 1.5); c- cabbage white butterfly (*P. brassicae*) showing abnormal (top) vs normal pupa (bottom) (× 1.5) (Adopted from (Mordue (Luntz) and Nisbet, (2000).

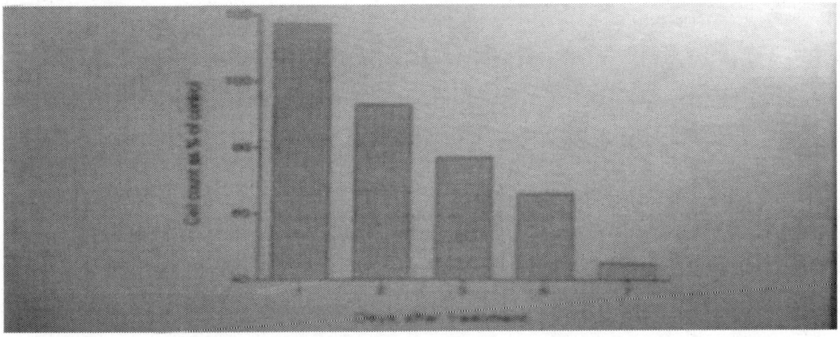

Figure 4. Inhibition of Spodoptera Sf9 cell proliferation after treatment with 10μM azadirachtin. (Sf9 cells were cultured in Graces cultured medium, supplemented with FCS. Azadirachtin was added in DMSO, final concentration1% and cell numbers were counted at 24 h intervals thereafter). (Adopted from Mordue (Luntz) and Nisbet, (2000).

NEEM SEED OIL TRIALS CARRIED OUT ON SPECIFIC PESTS

Pests of Soybean (*Glycine Max* (L.) Merrill)

Application of the Neem based formulations effectively controlled insect pests of Soybean (Naik, 2006) and Soybean borer and thrips (Stanley, 2010). Spraying 0.03% of the neem oil was found effective and caused 47% reduction in Soybean borer infestation (Rajabaskar, 2013). The Neem oil suspension at 0.5% sprayed on the lower surface of the leaf is very effective in controlling the population of whitefly nymphs (Naik, 2006). The treatment of Soybean seeds at different rates with the neem seed oil during planting did not produce any significant effect on the percentage emergency of Soybean. The height of the plants showed remarkable increase at a higher dose rate of 90 ml per one liter of water at 12 weeks after planting compared with control and other rates (Table 5). The Neem oil reduced pest attack on the crop and also defoliation of leaves which enhanced the leaf area that was necessary for the photosynthesis and proper growth of the crop. Besides, the Neem extracts contain hormones such as saponins and polyphenols which are active compounds that can stimulate the growth and yield of a plant (Andresen and Cedergreen, 2010). Thus in the similar work carried out by Okunlola and Ofuya, (2013) the Neem application increased the growth and yield of maize, soybean and jute in comparison to control. To actually ascertain the efficacy of the Neem oil, the population of insect pests was monitored through visual inspection and counting during their vegetative, flowering and podding stages of the soybean crop. Higher application of the Neem seed oil was noticed to have reduced the population of the major pests monitored (plates 4-12) at each phenology of the crop (Table 6). Severe infestation of insect on soybean plant caused defoliation and stunting of plant. As a result, the quality of the seed and yield decreased.

Table 5. Effect of the Neem Seed Oil on % Germination and Plant Height of Soybean (*Glycine max*)

	% germ.		Mean plant height (cm)				
Neem oil	*2WAP	2WAP	4WAP	6WAP	8WAP	10WAP	12WAP
0 ml	82.60	4.70	9.91	23.03	27.73	32.52	45.84
30	84.00	4.22	11.33	26.56	29.06	39.93	50.61
60	77.10	5.09	12.23	25.83	30.71	40.3	50.72
90	82.80	5.05	11.34	31.86	35.44	42.95	59.27
LSD0.05	NS	NS	1.42	0.82	0.93	0.52	1.31

*WAP –Weeks after planting.

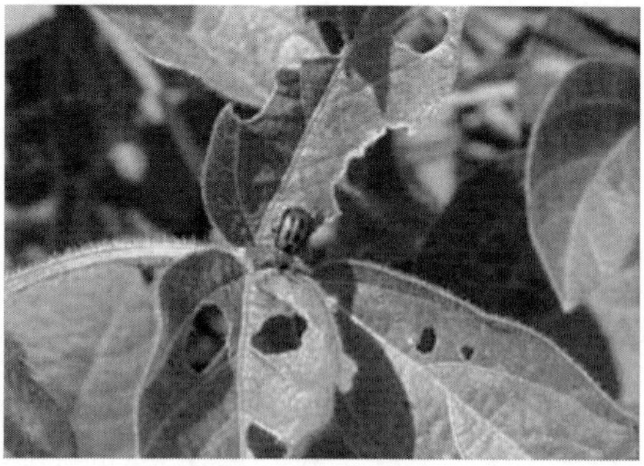

Plate 4. Bean Leaf Beetle.

Table 6. Effect of the Neem Oil on Insect Population of Soybean at Various Stages of Development

	Mean insect population at vegetative stage				Mean insect population at flowering stage				Mean insect population at podding stage		
Neem oil	2WAP	3WAP	4WAP	5WAP	6WAP	7WAP	8WAP	9WAP	10WAP	11WAP	12WAP
0ml	0.12	0.63	0.83	1.00	1.21	1.13	1.08	1.25	1.25	1.33	0.79
30ml	0.17	0.63	0.63	0.79	0.77	0.71	0.80	0.75	0.89	0.89	0.54
60ml	0.08	0.38	0.49	0.54	1.00	0.63	0.51	0.63	0.67	0.67	0.25
90ml	0.13	0.29	0.33	0.54	0.63	0.58	0.43	0.38	0.36	0.21	0.22
LSD 0.05	NS	NS	0.23	NS	0.18	0.49	0.37	0.48	0.41	0.38	0.38

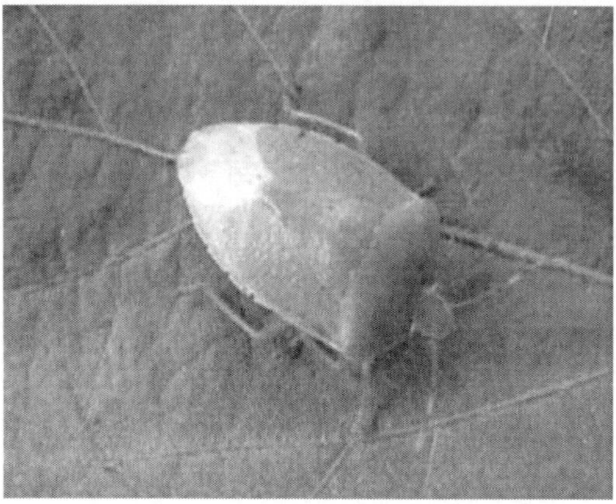

Plate 5. Green Stink Bug (*Nezara viridula*).

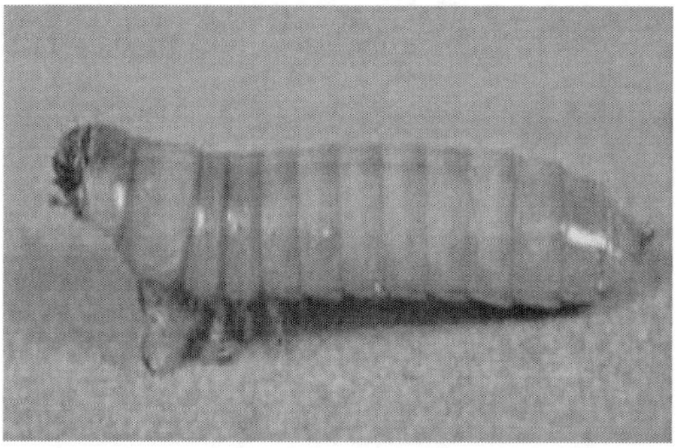

Plate 6. Large False.

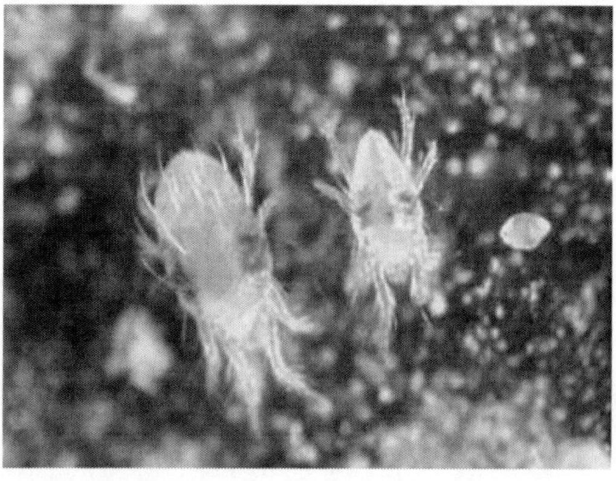

Plate 7.Two-Spotted Spider Mite.

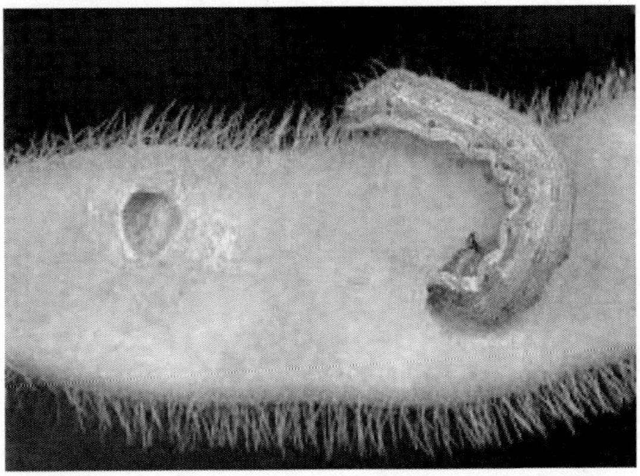

Plate 8. African Bollworm.

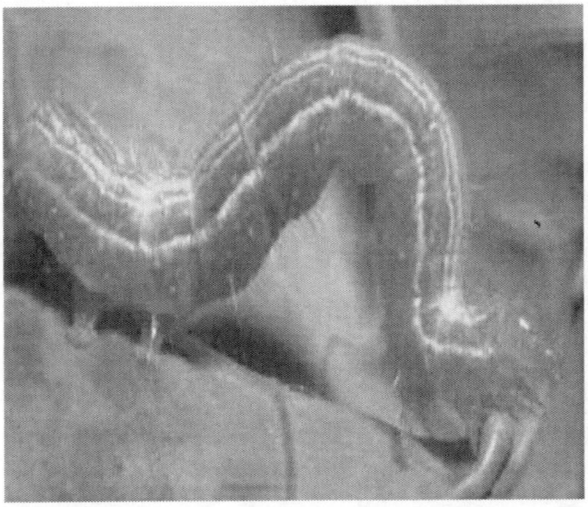

Plate 9. Cabbage Semi hopper.

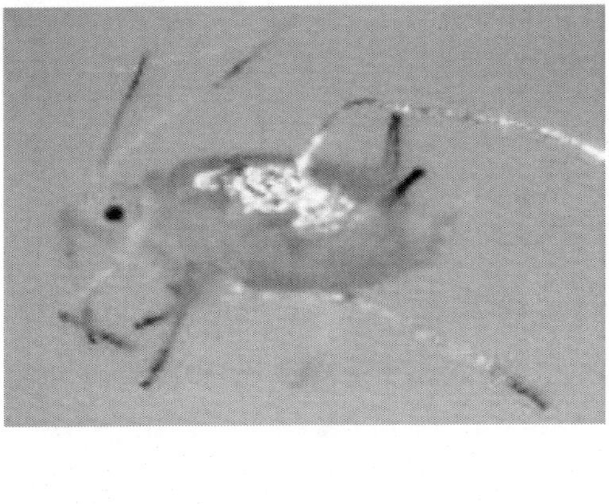

Plate 10. Aphids.

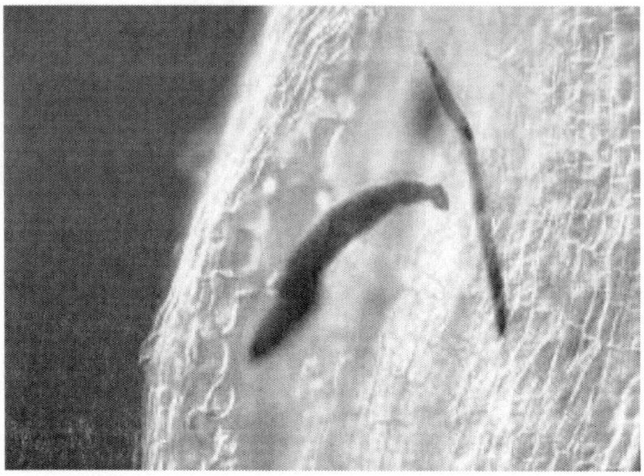

Plate 11. Soybean Cyst nematode.

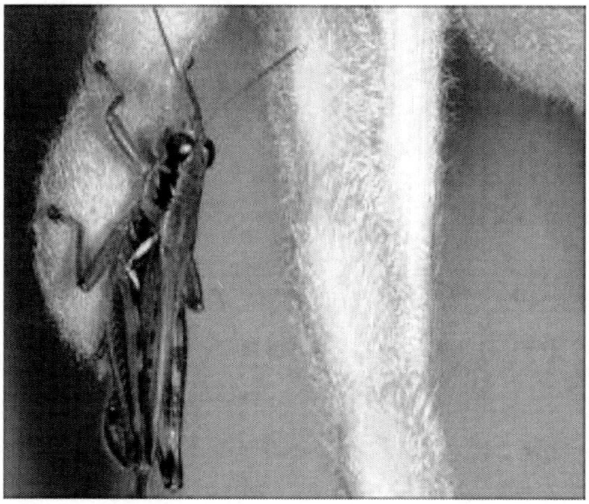

Plate 12. Grasshopper.

Pests of Okra

Okra plants botanically referred to as *Abelmoschus, esculentus* (L.), Moench, Several species of pests attack Okra. Most importantly, the podagrica species (plates 15, a-c) cause serious damage to the leaves by creating circular holes which invariably reduces the leaf area index, the photosynthetic ability and the pod production. Other Insects' such as white flies (plate 13), and cotton stainer (plate 16) were also seen also destroying the okra plants by attacking the flowers, pods, and stalks and thus cause the okra to fall prey to pathogenic organisms. Schmutterer (1995) also confirmed the potency of products from neem, *A. indica* tree for the control of field insect pests of egg plants and okra. The population of flea beetles on okra plant was properly managed by spraying oil extract from different parts of the neem tree (riped neem seed, unripe neem seed, and neem leaves) (Table 7). Among the oil extracts the riped neem seed oil appeared to be more effective compared with other parts of neem tree. The concentration of the active ingredient-azadirachtin on the riped neem seeds was more in the riped seeds. This appeared to have inhibited the activities of the flea beetles hence lowered pod damage and increased pod yield compared with other neem parts. Due to their compositional complexity, the neem oil based products can act as antifeedants, growth regulators, sterilants, anti-oviposition agents, and repellents (Gonzalez-Coloma, et al. 2013).The Azadirachtin in riped Neem seeds do not kill the flea beetles immediately, but inhibit their feeding, repel and disrupt their growth and reproduction (Drew, (1992).

While you may observe an aphid feeding singly, most often they are seen in masses, covering succulent new shoot and pods (plate 14). Their long, slender mouth parts are used to pierce stems, leaves, and other tender plant parts and suck up plant liquids. Large colonies of feeding aphids can weaken plant growth, cause leaves to yellow, curl or drop early. Some species can distort plant stems or fruit or cause galls on stems, leaves or roots. While landscape plants can generally tolerate extensive feeding by aphids, they can cause more serious damage to annual crops through transmission of viral diseases. As aphids feed, they produce honeydew that attracts ants. In fact, many species of ants are so addicted to this sweet drink that they will protect the aphids from various predators and move them to new plants if the one they are on starts to wilt. Some ants even build small shelters over species that feed near the base of the plant, to keep root-aphids inside their own nests. Any honeydew which the ants don’t consume can end up supporting the growth of black sooty.

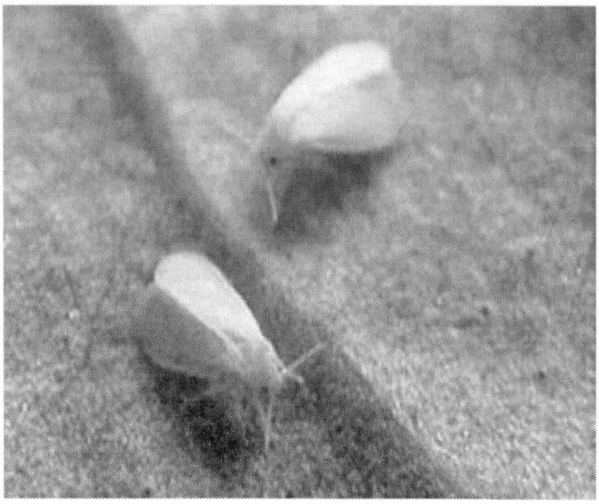

Plate 13. White Flies.

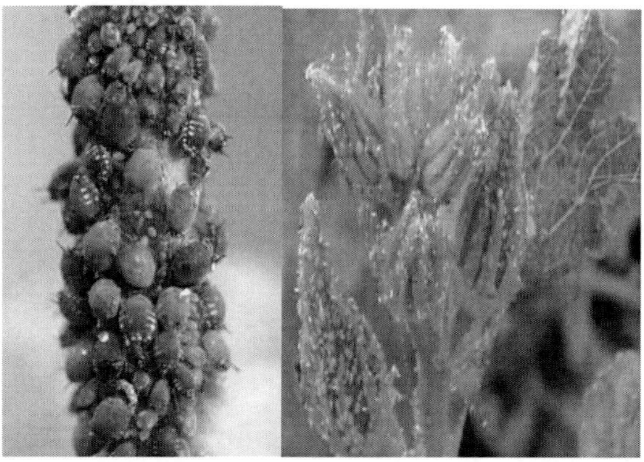

Plate 14. Aphids on Okra Pods.

Pests of Pigeonpea (*Cajanus cajan* (L.) Millsp is an important crop in semi-arid zones of the world. In Nigeria, the production of this crop is highly limited probably due to injurious effects of pests which are mostly abundant during the flowering phase (Dialoke et al. 2010). Sheldrake et al. (1979) in his work observed that pests that feed on the buds, flowers and pods have been implicated in the greatest economic damage. Hence, the population of leaf beetle, (*Aulacophora vinula* Eric) on pigeonpea flowers was high before spraying the Neem seed oil but after spraying with higher dosage of 6 ml per litre of water, the population was significantly reduced (Figures 5a, 6a, 7a, in April, 2009, May, 2010 and July 2010 (Dialoke et al.2015b). There was decreased population of *Riptortus dentipes* Fab. on improved pigeonpea pods after spraying a high dose of formulated Neem seed oil (F-NSO) at 6ml per litre on pigeonpea (Dialoke et al. 2014b). The okra flea beetles population (*podagrica* species) also decreased after spraying riped neem seed oil on okra plants compared with control (Dialoke et al., 2015a). The higher rate of F-NSO probably contained more active ingredients (*Azadirachtin*) and performed better than the lower rates.Better control of pests on pigeonpea was achieved using Neem and Tephrosia at higher concentrations (Kyamanywa et al. 2001).

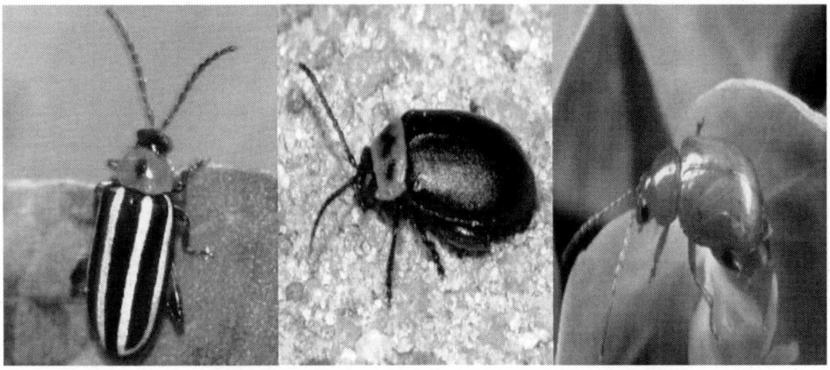

(a) (b) (c)

Plates 15. (a-c) Okra flea beetles (*podagrica* species).

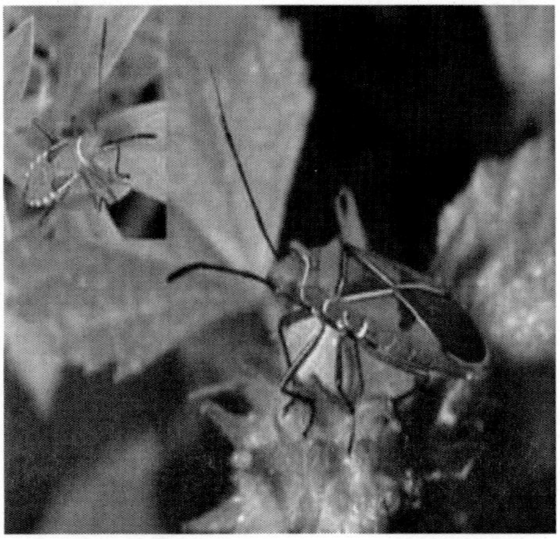

Plate 16. Cotton Stainer on Okra leaves.

Table 7. Effect of the Neem Oil on the Population of Podagrica spp, Damage and Yield (kg ha-1) of Okra Cultivar

Treatments	Population of *Podagrica* spp	Leaf damage by *Podagrica* spp	Green pod yield (g) per plant	Green pod yield (kg ha^{-1})
Control	24.44	52.60	0.81	54.00
Neem leaf oil	10.56	28.80	1.81	121.00
Ripped Neem				
Seed Oil	7.25	12.00	5.50	367.00
Unripped Neem				
Seed Oil	9.19	17.70	2.62	147.00
LSD 0.05	2.22	7.72	0.86	58.50
SE	3.14	10.9	1.22	82.20
CV (%)	24.5	39.3	45.5	48.0

Adopted from Dialoke et al. (2015a).

However, a weekly spraying F-NSO and synthetic pyrethroid (SPY) controlled the leaf beetle better than 2 or 3 weeks spraying (Figures 5b, 6b, 7b, (Dialoke et al. 2015b). Earlier studies on neem seed oil revealed that a weekly spraying of insecticides performed better than other spraying frequencies (Karungi et al. 2000; Dialoke et al.2014c).

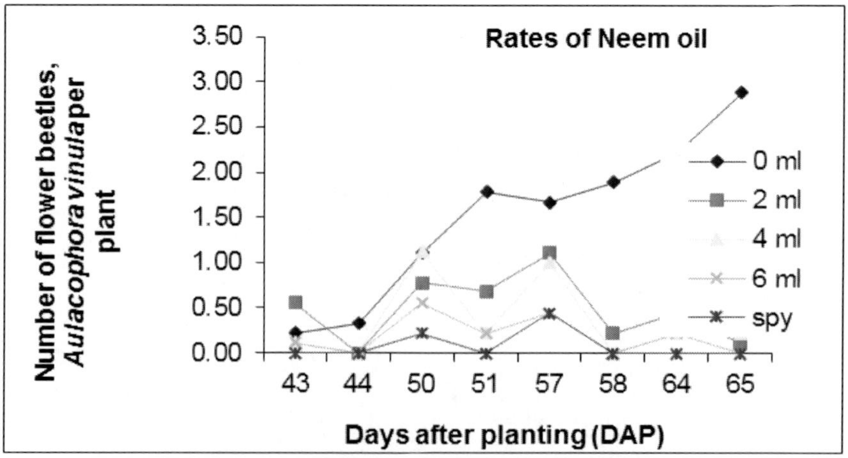

Figure 5 (a). The effect of the rates of Formulated Neem seed oil (F-NSO) and frequency of spraying on a number of flower beetles, *A. vinula* per plant during MAY 2009 planting season. (Adopted from Dialoke et al., 2015b).

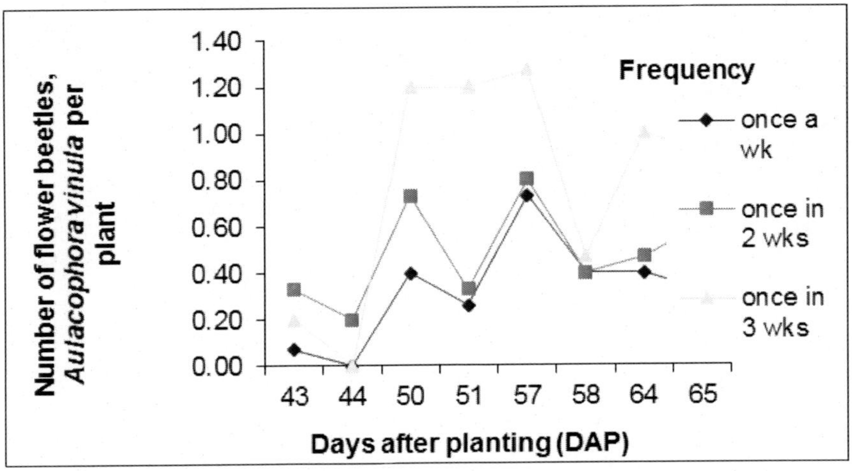

Figure 5 (b). The effect of frequency of spraying of formulated Neem seed oil (F-NSO) on a number of flower beetles, *A. vinula* per plant during MAY 2009 planting season. (Adopted from Dialoke et al., 2015b).

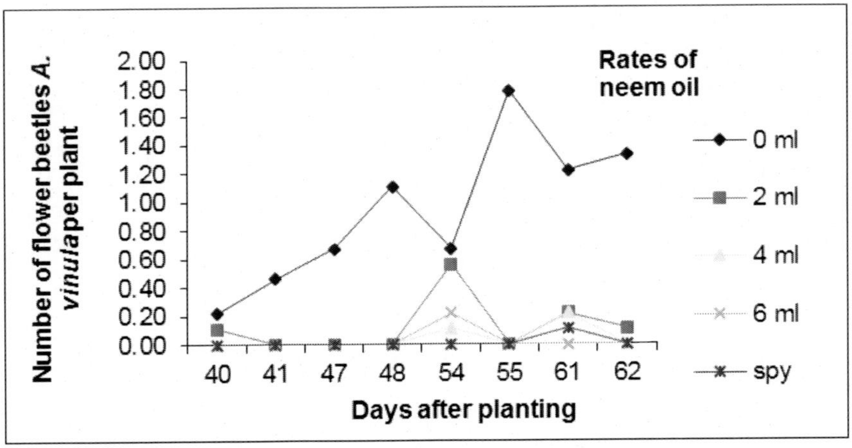

Figure 6 (a). The effect of the rates of formulated Neem seed oil (F-NSO) on a number of flower beetles, *A. vinula* per plant during MAY 2010 planting season. (Adopted from Dialoke et al., 2015b).

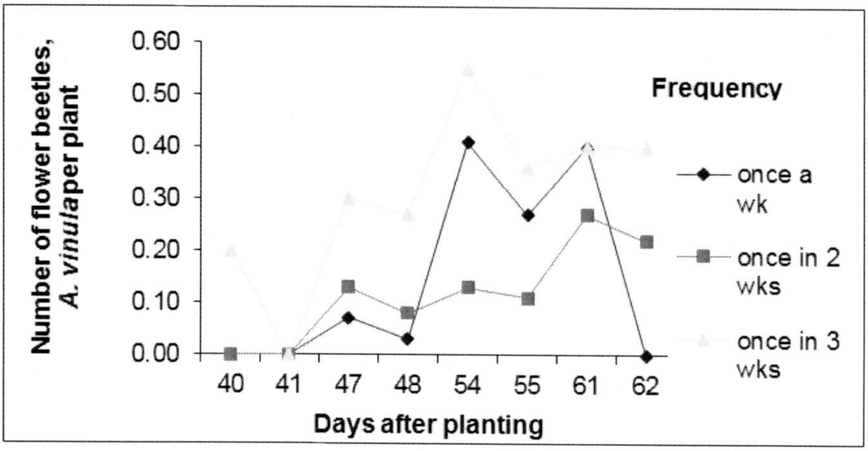

Figure 6(b). The effect of frequency of spraying of formulated Neem seed oil (F-NSO) on a number of flower beetles, *A. vinula* per plant during MAY 2010 planting season. (Adopted from Dialoke et al., 2015b).

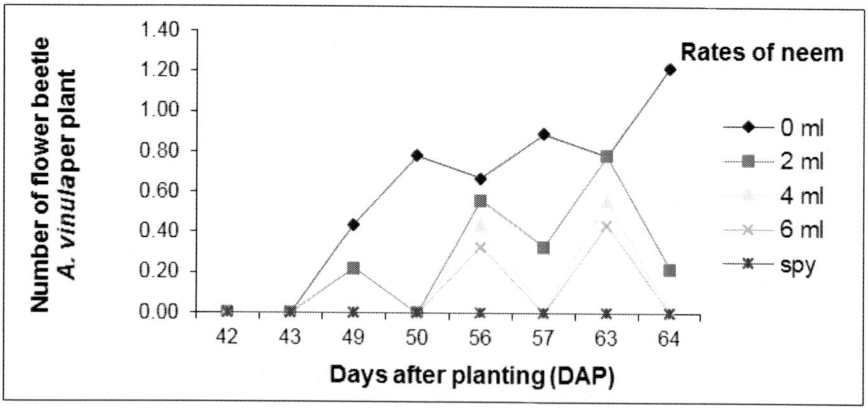

Figure 7 (a). The effect of the rates of formulated Neem seed oil (F-NSO) on a number of flower beetles, *A. vinula* per plant during July 2010 planting season. (Adopted from Dialoke et al., 2015b).

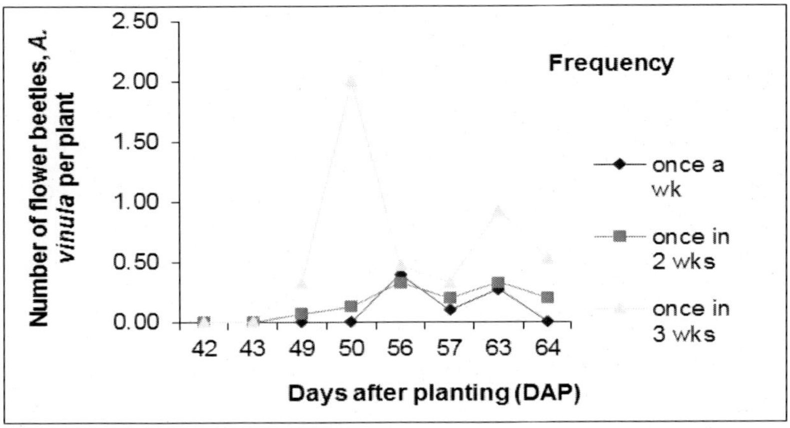

Figure 7 (b). The effect of frequency of spraying of formulated Neem seed oil (F-NSO) on a number of flower beetles, *A. vinula* per plant during July 2010 planting season. (Adopted from Dialoke et al., 2015b).

Podsucking Bugs Population and Damage on Pigeonpea

The presence of pod sucking bugs particularly the *R. dentipes* contributed to about 57.92-95.69% in kogi State, 59.71-80.85% in Benue State, and 68.50-93.10% in Imo State which subsequently limited the production of pigeonpea crops (Dialoke, et al. 2010). The adults and nymphs of *R. dentipes* fed on the developing pigeonpea pods. A high incidence of *R. dentipes* on pigeonpea pods in Owerri was earlier reported by Dialoke et al. (2014b). In all the planting seasons, (May, 2009, 2010 and July 2010) there was increased population of the *R. dentipes* before spraying the pods with the Neem seed oil and after spraying especially at a high dose of 6 ml/litre of water (12.5 ℓ in 840 litres of water ha^{-1}) Dialoke et al. (2014b). Their population drastically reduced while the population fluctuated in untreated pigeonpea plots in relation to days after spraying (Figures 8a, 9a, and 10a). This is a clear demonstration of the efficacy of the active ingredient, Azadirachtin in the Neem seed which has exerted repellent and antifeedant action against R. dentipes after spraying. Marco et al. (1990) research on pigeonpea also recorded ecdysteroid depletion when the Neem extracts were applied. The synthetic pyrethroid controlled the *R. dentipes* on the pods better than the F-NSO probably because of its contact poison activity. Moreover, the insecticidal activity of azadirachtin has been demonstrated against numerous other insect pests (Schmutterer and Singh, 1995, 2002, Oparaeke et al. 2006, Oparaeke, 2005; Basdove et al. 2002, Dialoke et al. 2014 c on thrips) and its various mode of action can include disruption of feeding, reproduction or development (Mordue (Luntz) et al. 1998 and Walter, 1999).

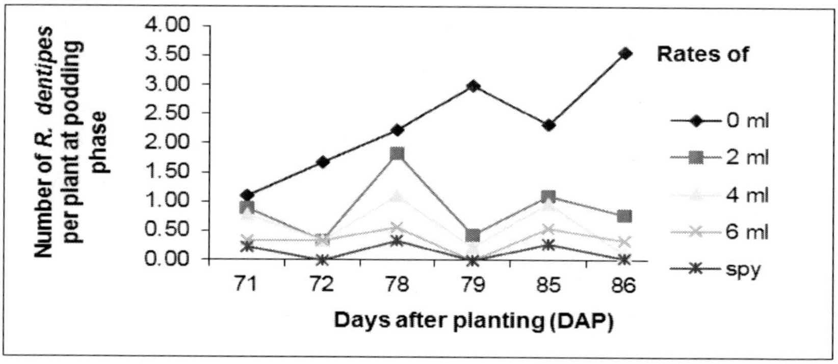

Dialoke et al.2014b.

Figure 8 (a). The effect of the rates of formulated Neem seed oil (F-NSO) on a number of *R. dentipes* per plant at podding phase during MAY 2009 planting season.

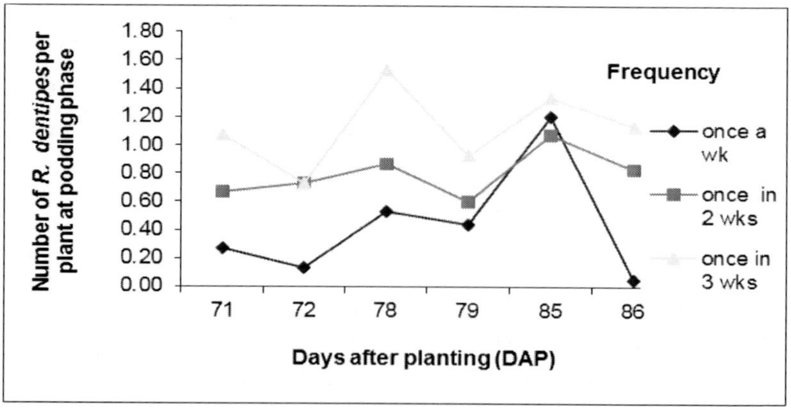

Dialoke et al.2014b.

Figure 8 (b). The effect of frequency of spraying of formulated Neem seed oil (F-NSO) on a number of *R. dentipes* per plant at podding phase during MAY 2009 planting season.

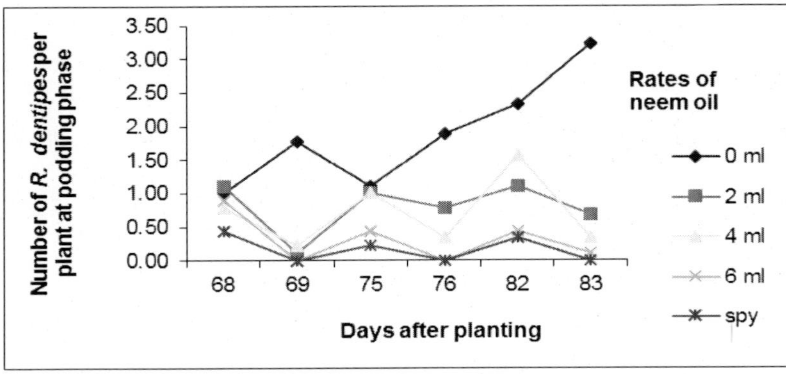

Dialoke et al.2014b.

Figure 9 (a). The effect of the rates of formulated Neem seed oil (F-NSO) on a number of *R. dentipes* per plant at podding phase during MAY 2010 planting season.

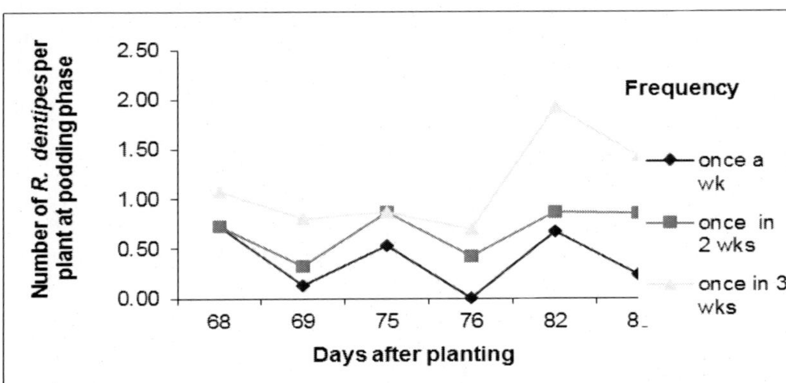

Dialoke et al.2014b.

Figure 9 (b). The effect of frequency of spraying of formulated Neem seed oil (F-NSO) on a number of *R. dentipes* per plant at podding phase during MAY 2010 planting season.

The Neem oil and the synthetic pyrethroids at a weekly spraying controlled the *R. dentipes* effectively but for economic reasons spraying at once in 2 weeks seems to be a more reasonable control of the pest when compared to spraying once in 3 weeks (Dialoke et al. (2014b; Degri and Hadi, 2002) (Figures 8b, 9b and 10b). The repellent activity of Azadirachtin in the Neem seed prevented the *R. dentipes* from feeding on the pods due to the presence of deterrent taste factors. Moreso *R. dentipes* stopped feeding at some point after ingestion the food due to secondary hormonal or physiological effects of the deterrent substances (Olaifa et al. 1991). Also the oil acts as a growth regulator which disrupts normal development and chitin synthesis of insects with the susceptibility to the potency of the neem differing from species to species, (Olaifa et al. 1991, Jackai and Oyediran, 1991).

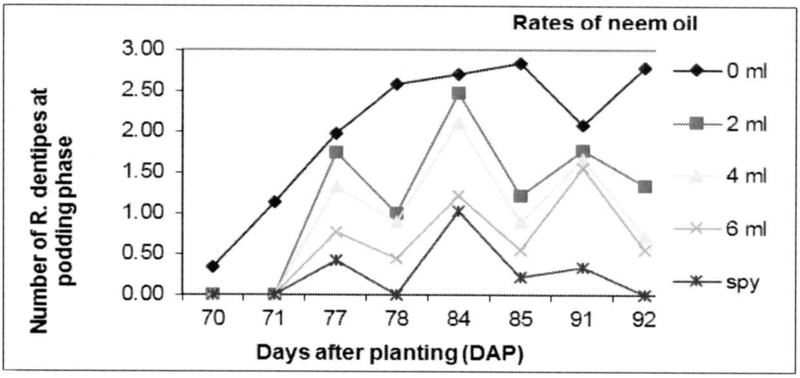

Dialoke et al.2014b.

Figure 10 (a). The effect of the rates of formulated Neem seed oil (F-NSO) on a number of *R. dentipes* per plant at podding phase during JULY 2010 planting Season.

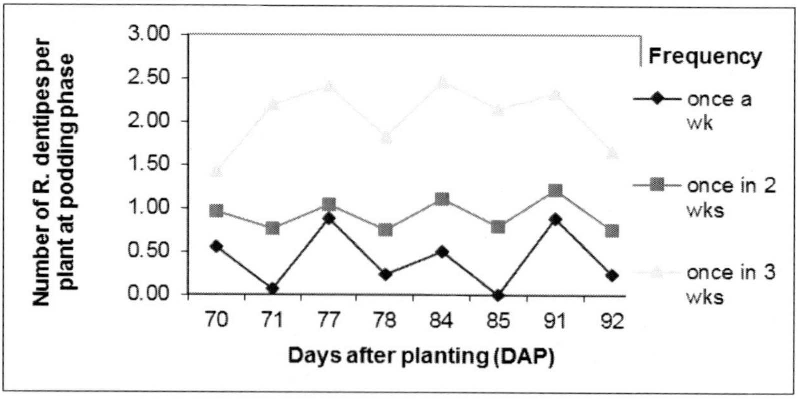

Dialoke et al.2014b.

Figure 10 (b). The effect of frequency of spraying of formulated Neem seed oil (F-NSO) on a number of *R. dentipes* per plant at podding phase during JULY 2010 planting season.

The Pigeonpea damage by these podsucking bugs: *Riptortus dentipes* Fab, *Nezara viridula* (L.) *Clavigralla tomentosicollis* Stal., *Clavigralla. shaddabi*Dolling,etc., have been reported as the major constraints to itsproduction in Nigeria (Dialoke et al.2010). Out of this entire podsucking bugs, the *R. dentipes* possess the greatest threat to pigeonpea production in Imo State as its population appears at all time of the cropping seasons (Dialoke et al. 2014a). Also, in a survey carried out on pigeonpea growing areas in Nigeria between February 2007 and 2008, the *R. dentipes* were identified in Imo state as the most pod damaging pests compared with all other states (Dialoke et al. 2010). Emosairue, (2007), in his research on cowpea reported these podsucking bugs complex namely: *C. tomentosicollis*, *A. curvipes, and Mirperus jaculus* as major insect pests that decimate cowpeas at their podding stage.

Assessment of Pods and Seeds Damage by Insect Pests

At maturity the pigeonpea pods were harvested and threshed manually. The pods and seeds were examined for insect damage and the incidence of damage assessed as the proportion of pods and seeds shriveled, twisted, and constricted. The Pod/Seed damage indices (Sdi), were determined by sorting the pod/seed from each plot into seeds with no feeding damage (wholesome pods/seeds), pods/seeds severely shrunken to small sizes (shriveled), and mild shrinkles. The proportions of each category from 100 pods/seeds selected at random from each plot were counted, and expressed as percentage of the total pods /seeds assessed, as shown below:

$$\text{Pod/Seed Damage (\%)} = \frac{\text{No.of Damaged Pods/Seeds}}{\text{Total No.of Pods/Seeds Examined}} \times \frac{10}{1}$$

$$\text{Pod/Seed Damage (\%)} = \frac{\text{No. of Damaged Pods/Seeds}}{\text{Total No. of Pods/Seeds Examined}} \times \frac{100}{1}$$

The percentage pod and seed damage by the *R. dentipes*, during May 2009, 2010 and July 2010 planting seasons, as well as percentage wholesome pods and seeds were influenced by different rates of the Neem seed oil (Table 8). The pigeonpea plants that were sprayed with the high dose of Neem seed oil recorded low percentage pods shriveled by the *R. dentipes* but were inferior to pigeonpea plots sprayed with synthetic pyrethroids (SPY). Similarly, the percentage wholesome pods and seeds were also higher than the control plots. Plates 17 shows the nature of damaged pods/seeds (a,b) by the *R. dentipes* and normal pods/seeds (c, d). In the field, the *R. dentipes* continually go into mating, producing young nymphs with overwhelming population especially during early morning sun and evening weather (plate 17e). The spraying of the Neem seed oil at once a week, recorded the least percentage pods shriveled and greater portion of wholesome pods and seeds.

The lowest percentage pods and seeds damages were recorded during July planting season compared with May 2009 and 2010 planting seasons. The bitter taste of Azadirachtin in the Neem seed oil deterred the *R. dentipes* from feeding (sucking sap from flowers and young pods) and thus gave rise to low pod and seed shriveled. There was an increased percentage of wholesome pods/seeds quality. The unprotected plots recorded a greater percentage of pods and seeds damage given rise to the lowest percentage of wholesome pods and seeds compared with protected plots. However, the plots sprayed with synthetic pyrethroid (SPY) were much better protected than plots sprayed with the neem seed oil (F-NSO) and untreated (control) plots. The synthetic insecticide is a contact insecticide which has caused quick mortality to the *R. dentipes* pests in contact with the spraying liquids hence the efficacy was higher than spraying with the Neem seed oil. However, the application of the Neem seed oil at weekly intervals recorded the least percentage of pod/seeds damage as well as the highest percentage of wholesome pods and seeds followed by once in two weeks or at least with once in three weeks application. This implies that the application of the insecticides at once in three weeks could not have effective control over the *R. dentipes* population during the podding phase of the early maturing stages of the pigeonpea. The short residual activity of the Azadirachtin and the synthetic pyrethroid often made the spray liquids not to stay effectively on the plants longer than three weeks. Furthermore, the changes in climatic conditions played a significant role to the pods/seeds damage which was experienced more in May 2009, followed by 2010 and the least during July 2010 planting season.

Pods and Seeds Damaged by Podsucking Bugs

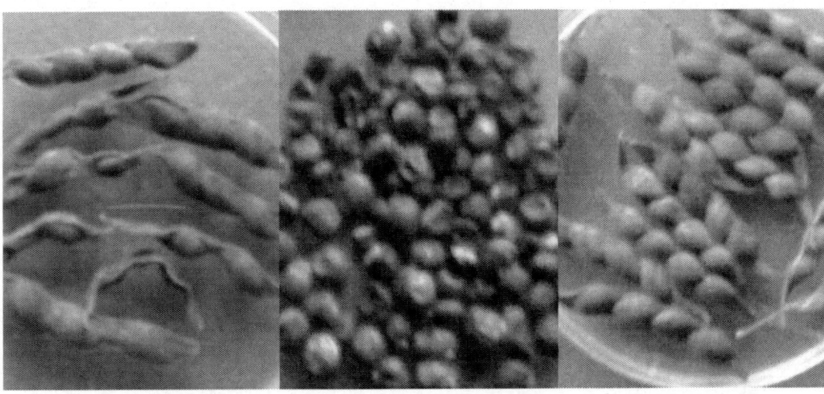

(a) Shriveled pods (b) shriveled seeds (c) wholesome pods

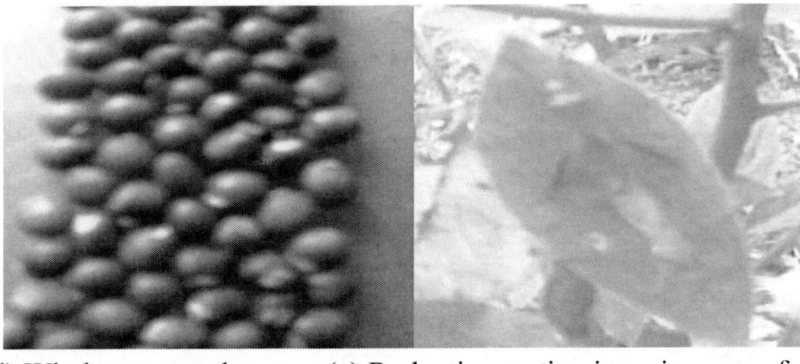

(d) Wholesome seeds (e) R. dentipe mating in a pigeonpea farm

Plates 17.

The Effect of the Different Rates of Formulated Neem Seed Oil (F-NSO) and the Frequency of Application on the *R. dentipes* Damage of Early Maturing Pigeonpea Cultivar at Different Planting Seasons in Owerri

	May 2009				May 2010				July 2010			
Rates of Neem oil (NO)	% pods shriveled by *R.dentipes*	% seeds shriveled by *R.dentipes*	% whole-some pods	% whole-some seeds	% pods shriveled by *R.dentipes*	% seeds shriveled by *R.dentipes*	% whole-some pods	% wholesome seeds	% pods shriveled by *R.dentipes*	% seeds shriveled by *R. dentipes*	% whole-some pods	% whole-some seeds
0 ml (0 ℓha^{-1})	97.80	9.30	2.20	0.70	51.70	85.91	3.40	8.20	36.48	49.00	59.22	45.70
2 ml (4.2 ℓha^{-1})	73.20	84.70	16.26	9.52	36.20	72.00	27.90	26.00	29.56	47.00	68.56	52.90
4 ml (8.3 ℓha^{-1})	65.50	76.40	28.24	21.14	33.90	66.90	36.10	31.43	27.22	44.60	71.00	53.60
6 ml (12.5 ℓha^{-1})	55.60	60.40	40.40	37.93	28.10	52.10	45.90	47.60	24.23	38.60	74.44	58.30
SPY (1.5 ℓha^{-1})	42.60	37.69	55.73	62.20	17.00	34.60	71.40	65.30	18.11	27.30	81.56	73.80
LSD 0.05	12.20	8.66	12.90	8.23	6.61	11.73	8.88	12.06	5.27	7.90	5.16	6.92

	May 2009				May 2010				July 2010			
Frequency (F)												
Once a week	57.80	63.96	36.59	33.10	29.60	56.30	44.60	42.50	24.96	32.90	73.60	67.10
% pods shriveled	% seeds shriveled	% whole-some	% whole-some	% pods shriveled	% seeds shriveled	% whole-some	% whole-ome	% pods shriveled	% seeds shriveled	% whole-some	% whole-some	
by *R.dentipes*	*by R.dentipes*	pods	seeds	by *R.dentipes*	*by R.dentipes*	pods	seeds	by *R.dentipes*	*by R.dentipes*	pods	seeds	
Once in 2 wks	64.00	67.80	28.38	28.00	32.60	60.90	37.50	37.17	26.47	36.60	71.80	63.40
Once in 3 wks	68.80	77.73	19.20	17.40	37.90	69.10	28.80	28.10	29.27	54.70	68.13	40.70
LSD 0.05	N.S	6.71	9.99	6.38	5.12	9.08	6.88	9.34	4.09	6.12	3.99	5.36
interaction												
(NO × F.)	N.S	15.00	N.S	14.26	N.S	N.S	N.S	N.S	N.S	N.S	N.S	N.S

Population Dynamics of Thrips on Pigeonpea Crops

The pigeonpea plants is prone to flower thrips (*Megalurothrips usitatus* Bagnall) (plate 18) infestation causing considerable losses to flowers of pigeonpea (Kimani, 1987). The damage by thrips in early stages of pigeonpea crop growth is more important and would likely result to substantial reduction in its yield (Raheja (1973). Thrips can also act as vectors of viral diseases on pigeonpea. Several control measures have been advocated. They include cultural, use of resistant varieties and insecticides. However, these interventions have not been able to solve the problems of thrips on the farmers' fields. Presently, insecticides are the only method for the effective control of thrips for a reasonable pod yields (Jackai and Adalla, 1997).

Thus in a research carried out at Owerri in May 2009, 2010 and July, 2010, the application of the neem seed oil had no effect on the population of flower thrips even at higher dosage rate of 6 ml per litre of water but they were reduced with the application of synthetic pyrethroids (Figures 11a, 12a, and 13a).The synthetic pyrethroid had contact toxicity and could penetrate the inside flowers to kill hidden thrips better than the neem seed oil that had very low contact activity which could not penetrate the flowers to locate the thrips (Dialoke et al. 2014 c). Spraying intervals had no effect on the thrips (Figures 11b, 12b, and 13b).

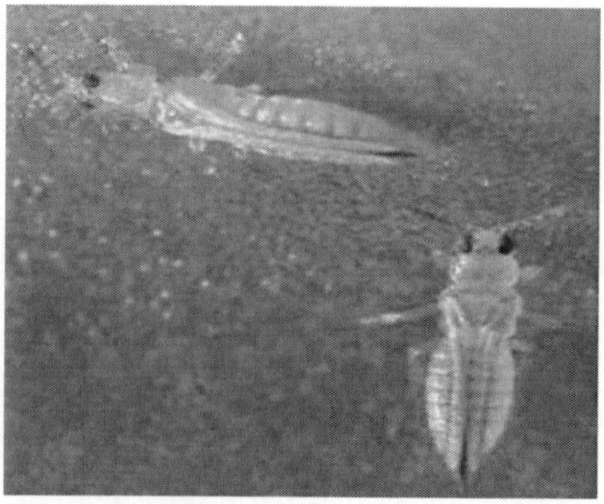

Plate 18. Flower thrips.

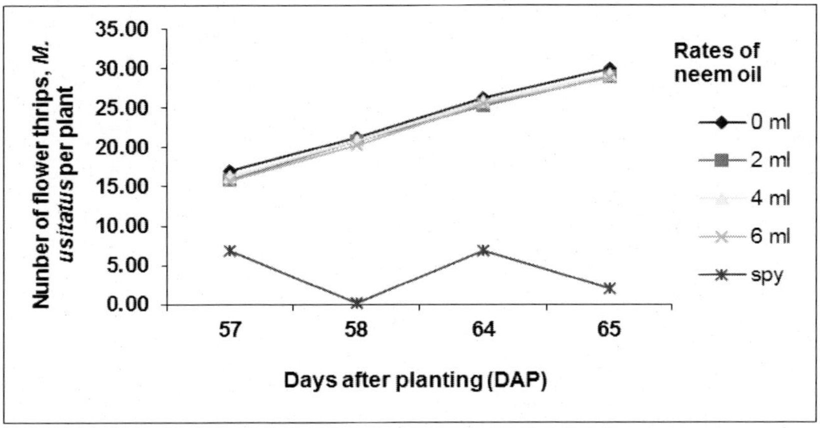

Dialoke, et al. 2014 c.

Figure 11 (a). The effect of the rates of formulated Neem seed oil (F-NSO) on a number of flower thrips, *M. usitatus* per plant at flowering phase during MAY 2009 planting season.

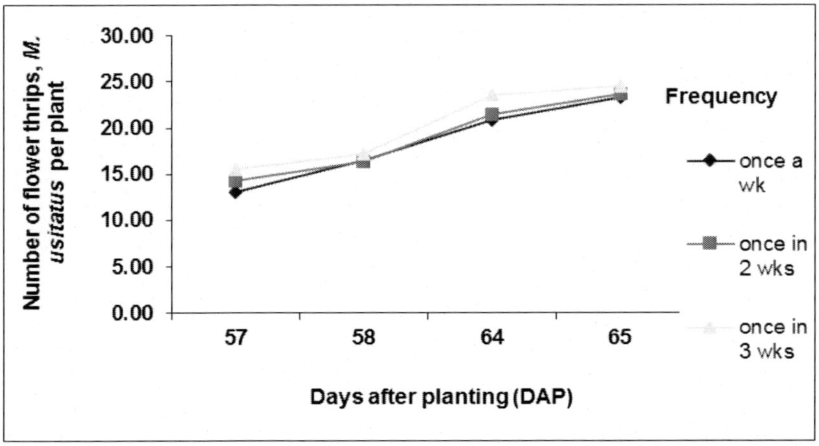

Dialoke, et al. 2014 c.

Figure 11 (b). The effect of frequency of spraying of formulated Neem seed oil (F-NSO) on a number of flower thrips, *M. usitatus* per plant at flowering phase during MAY 2009 planting season.

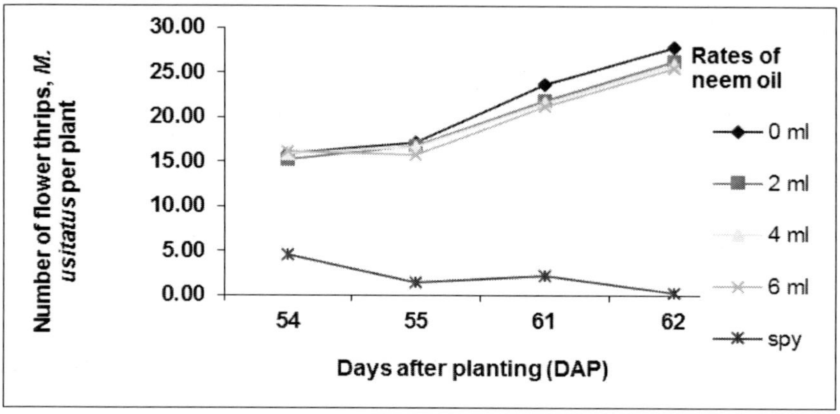

Dialoke, et al. 2014 c.

Figure 12 (a). The effect of the rates of formulated Neem seed oil (F-NSO) on a number of flower thrips, *M. usitatus* per plant at flowering phase during MAY 2010 planting season.

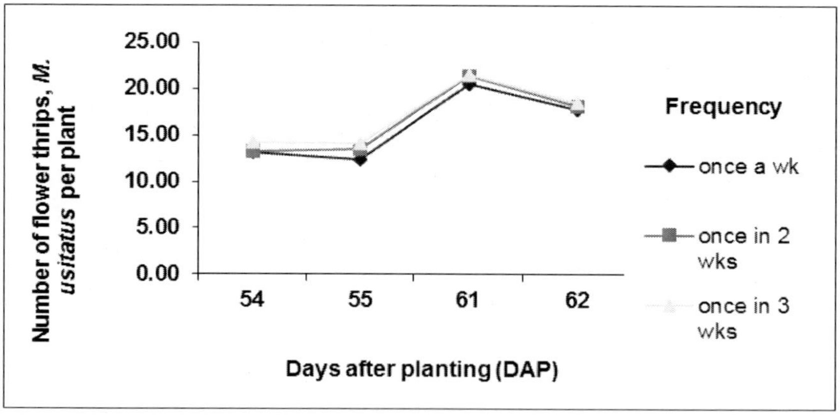

Dialoke, et al. 2014 c.

Figure 12 (b). The effect of frequency of Spraying of formulated Neem seed oil (F-NSO) on a number of flower thrips, *M. usitatus* per plant at flowering phase during MAY 2010 planting season.

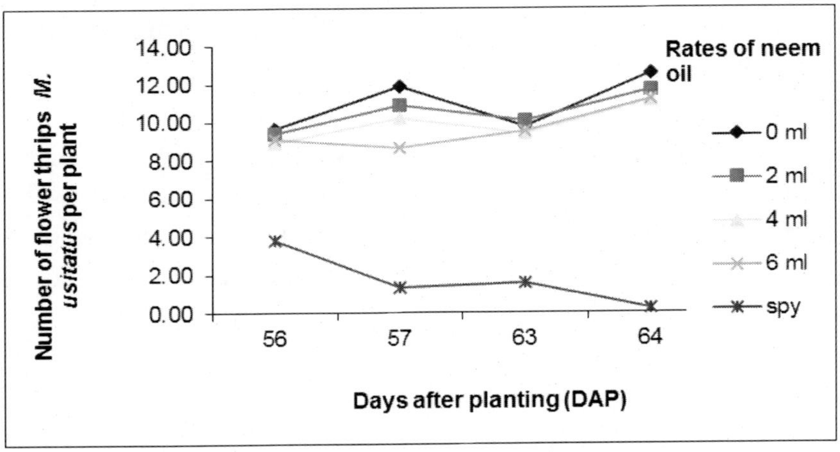

Dialoke, et al. 2014 c.

Figure 13 (a). The effect of the rates of formulated Neem seed oil (F-NSO) on a number of flower thrips, *M. usitatus* per plant at flowering phase during JULY 2010 planting season.

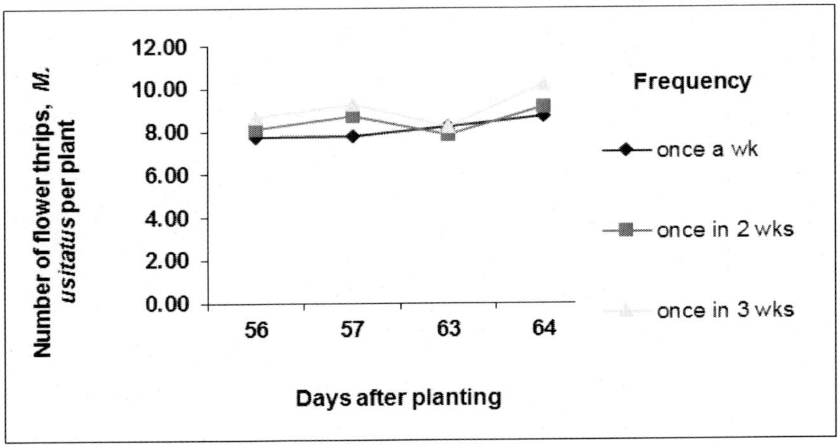

Dialoke, et al. 2014 c.

Figure 13 (b). The effect of frequency of spraying of formulated Neem seed oil (F-NSO) on a number of flower thrips, *M. usitatus* per plant at flowering phase during JULY 2010 planting season.

Researches Information on Podborer Population and Damage to Pigeonpea Crops

The podborer: *Helicoverpa armigera* Hubner and *Maruca vitrata* Fab have been the major problems of pigeonpea production all over the pigeonpea growing area of sub-Saharan continent of the world (Manjunath et al.1995 in India, Dialoke et al. 2010; Dialoke, 2017 in Nigeria and kimani, 1987 in Kenya). The infestation is responsible for heavy loss in early and medium late maturing pigeonpea genotypes (Sahoo, 1995; Shanower et al. 1999). The young larvae of the legume podborer feeds mainly on flowers and young pods of different plants (Chi et al. 2003; Rekha and Mallapur, 2007) while the mature larvae feeds on pods (Liao and Lin, 2000). The third and 5th instar larvae are capable of boring into the pigeonpea pods and can consume the developing grains (Gopali et al. 2010). The population of *Helicoverpa armigera* Hubner (plate 21), on pigeonpea pods before spraying was very high in the months of May 2009, 2010 and July 2010 but soon after spraying with the Neem seed oil at the dosage rate of 6 ml/litre of water (12.5ℓ in 840 litres of water ha^{-1}), the population got reduced. The synthetic pyrethroid still performed better than the control and Neem seed oil treated plots (Figures 14a, 15a, and 16a). The population of the legume pod borer, *Maruca vitrata* at weekly spraying intervals with high dose of crude seed extract of Neem and mahogany plants at 150 g per litre of water was controlled (Rouf and Sardar 2011). Most often, the pigeonpea, maize, and chickpea had high population of pod borers in the untreated plots than the plots treated with the neem seed oil (Night and Ogenga-latigo (1994), Nourai (1987), Al-dabei et al. (2007) Khurana (1997). Application of water extract from the Neem seed and kernel on potted cowpea plants controlled, the podborer,and *Maruca testulalis* (IITA, 1993); Kyamanywa et al. 2001). The Azadirachtin in formulated Neem seed oil (F-NSO) exerted not only repellent but antifeedant effects on the *H. armigera*. Again, the respiratory pores of the *H. armigera* with a gas exchange were blocked by the neem seed oil which resulted to the death of the pod borer.

The synthetic pyrethroid attacks the neurosecretory cells of *H. arimigera* thereby disrupting the balance of neurohormones within the insect and this accounts for its potency in the control of the pest compared to the Neem seed oil (Henrick, 1995). However, the application of Neem seed oil at once a week had a better control of the population of *H. armigera* compared with other intervals of application (Figure 14b,15b and 16b) (Dialoke, 2017). With respect to damage across the planting seasons, the percentage of pod/seed damage of formulated neem seed oil (F-NSO) increased as the rates increased from 2-6ml/litre of water compared with the untreated control but proved less effective compared with synthetic pyrethroid (Table 9). Some factors like low concentration of the Neem seed oil, non- persistence on the leaves and dilution with rainfall affected the performance of the neem seed oil when compared with the synthetic pyrethroid (Dialoke, 2017). A range of 13.58-84.28% and 3.15-84.28% damage respectively occurred to pods and seeds of chickpea, *Cicer arietinum* L., by pod borer (Joginder et al. 1990). In favourable conditions the pod damage can be as high as 90.95 percent (Shengal and Ujagir,1990; Sachan and Katti, 1994). On the average, 30 to 40 percent of chickpea *Cicer arietinum* L. pods were found to be damaged by pod borer areas in Bangladesh with an average of 400 kg ha^{-1} grain loss (Rahman, 1990; Begum et al. 1992), Lal, (1996), King and Sawicki, (1990).

Intervals of application at once a week consistently recorded the lowest pod damage by *H. armigera* throughout the planting seasons compared with application of once in two or three weeks (Figure 13b, 14b and 15b) (Dialoke, 2017). The July 2010, season had the least percentage of pod and seed damage, with feeding holes and punctures (plates 19, a-b). This protection potentials of the Neem seed oil enhanced better quality of pods and seeds (wholesome pods/seeds (plates 20, a-b). Hence, the July planting season appeared to be the best period for planting the short duration pigeonpea in Owerri agro-ecological rainforest zone of Southeastern, Nigeria.

Pods and Seeds Damaged by *H. armigera*

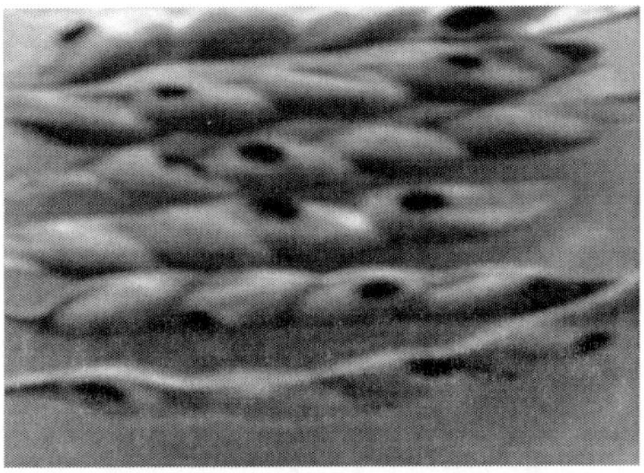

Plate 19 (a). Pods bored by *H. armigera.*

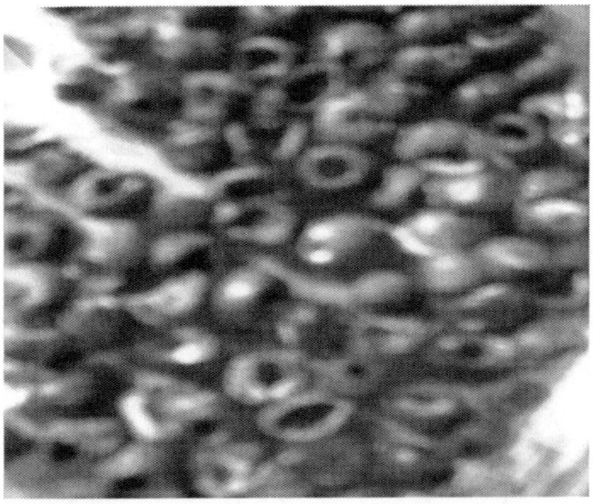

Plate (b).Seeds bored by *H. armigera.*

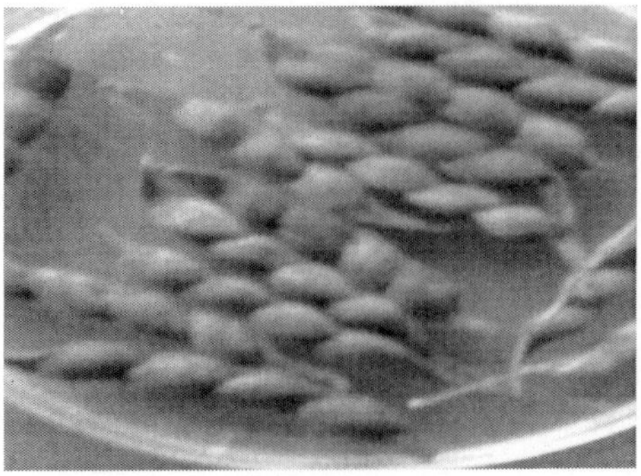

Plate20 (a). Wholesome pods.

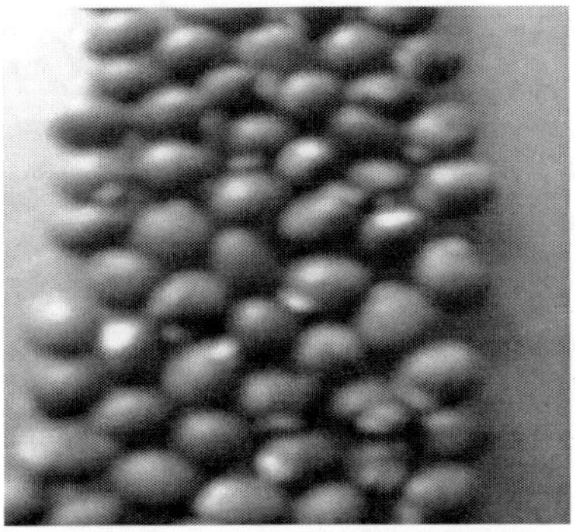

Plate(b). Wholesome seeds.

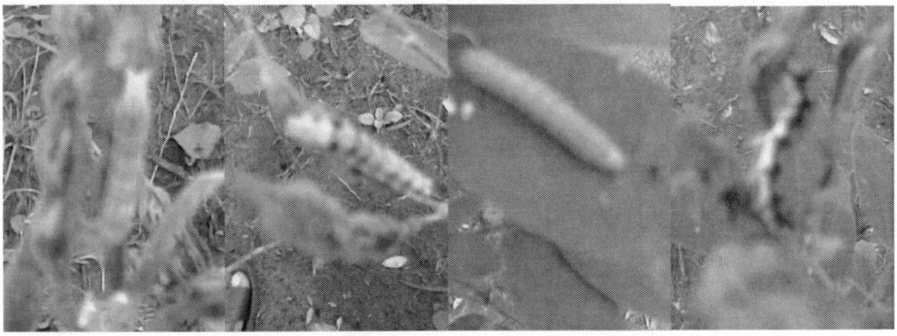

Plate 21. Pod borer complex (*Helicoverpa armigera*) damaging pigeonpea pods arranged in colours.

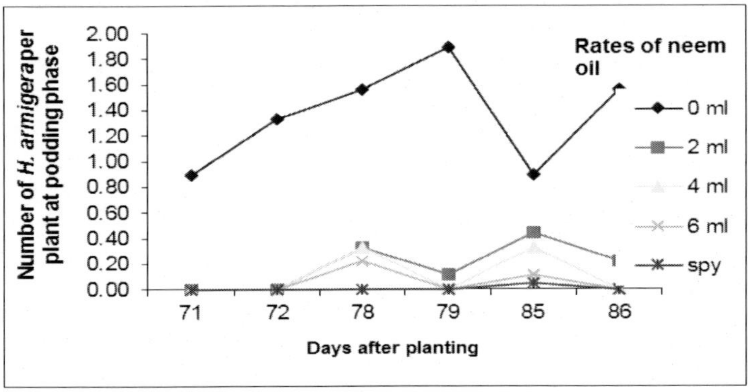

Dialoke, 2017.

Figure 14 (a). The effect of the rates of F-NSO on a number of *H. armigera* per plant at podding phase during MAY 2009 planting season.

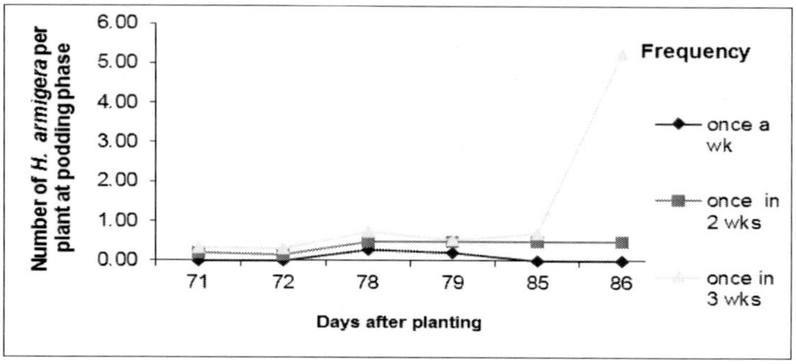

Dialoke, 2017.

Figure 14 (b). The effect of frequency of spraying of F-NSO on a number of *H. armigera* per plant at podding phase during MAY 2009 planting season.

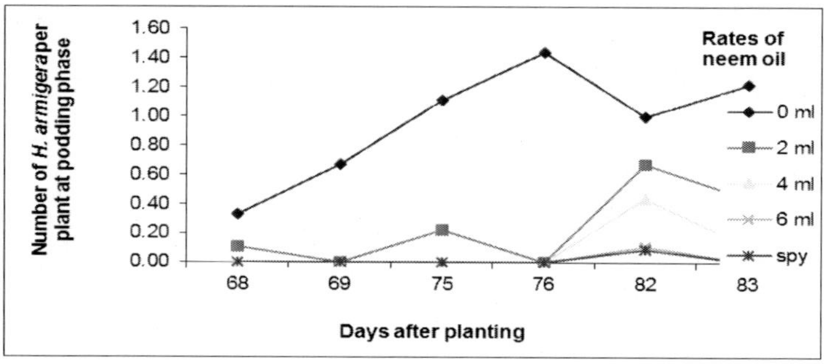

Dialoke, 2017.

Figure 15 (a).The effect of the rates of F-NSO on a number of *H. armigera* per plant at podding phase during MAY 2010 planting season.

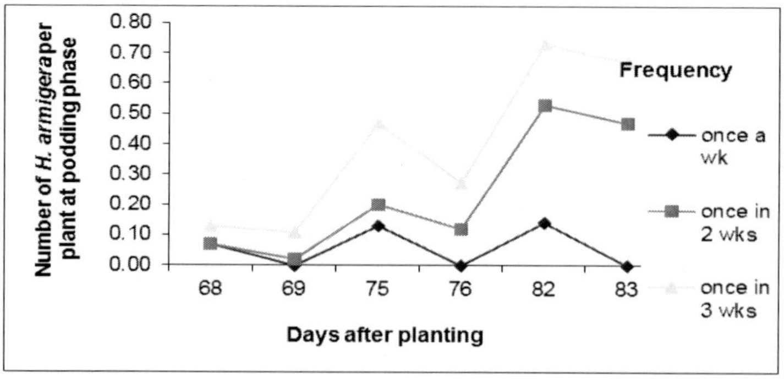

Dialoke, 2017.

Figure 15 (b). The effect of frequency of spraying of F-NSO on a number of *H. armigera* per plant at podding phase during MAY2010 planting season.

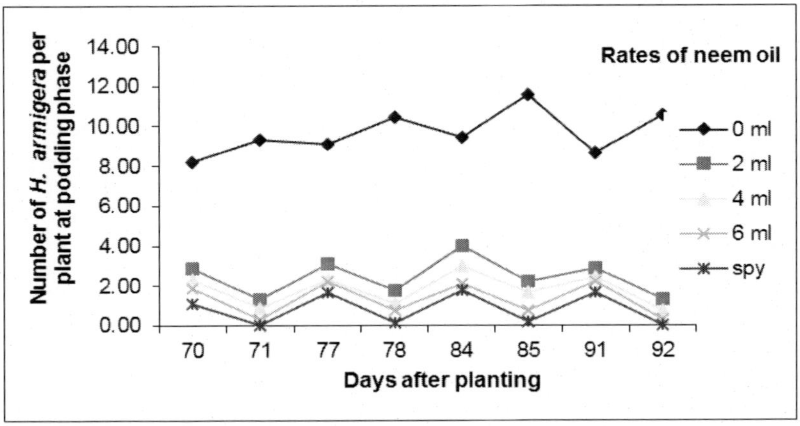

Dialoke, 2017.

Figure 16 (a). The effect of the rates of F-NSO on a number of *H. armigera* per plant at podding phase during JULY 2010 planting season.

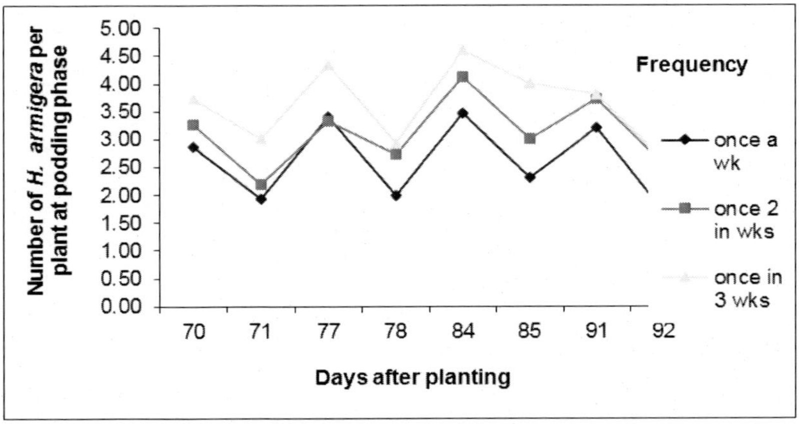

Dialoke, 2017.

Figure 16 (b). The effect of frequency of spraying of F-NSO on a number of *H. armigera* per plant at podding phase during JULY 2010 planting season.

Table 9. The effects of the rates and application frequency of F-NSO on the *H. armigera* population and the damage of early maturing pigeonpea cultivar in Owerri, Nigeria

	MAY-2009				**MAY-2010**				**JUL-2010**			
Rates of Neem (NO)	% pods bored by *H. armigera*	% seeds bored by *H. armigera*	% wholesome pods	% wholesome seeds	% pods bored by *H. armigera*	% seeds bored by *H. armigera*	% wholesome pods	% wholesome seeds	% pods bored by *H. armigera*	% seeds bored by *H. armigera*	% wholesome pods	% wholesome seeds
0 ml (0 ℓha^{-1})	16.35	10.00	2.90	0.70	44.90	5.89	3.40	8.20	4.30	0.00	59.22	45.70
2 ml (4.2 ℓ ha^{-1})	10.54	5.78	16.26	9.52	35.90	2.00	27.90	26.00	1.89	0.00	68.56	52.90
4 ml (8.3 ℓha^{-1})	6.26	2.46	28.24	21.14	30.00	1.67	36.10	31.43	1.78	0.00	71.00	53.60
6 ml (12.5 ℓ ha^{-1})	4.00	1.67	40.40	37.93	26.00	0.33	45.90	47.60	1.33	0.00	74.44	58.30
SPY (1.5 ℓha^{-1})	1.67	0.11	55.73	62.20	11.60	0.11	71.40	65.30	0.33	0.00	81.56	73.80
LSD 0.05	3.68	2.62	12.90	8.23	6.68	1.97	8.88	12.06	1.02	N.S	5.16	6.92
Frequency (F)												
Once a week	5.61	2.94	36.59	33.10	25.80	1.27	44.60	42.5	1.44	0.00	73.6	67.10
Once in 2 wks	7.62	4.20	28.38	28.00	29.90	1.93	37.50	37.17	1.73	0.00	71.8	63.40

	MAY-2009				**MAY-2010**				**JUL-2010**			
Rates of Neem	% pods bored	% seeds bored	% wholesome	% wholesome	% pods bored	% seeds bored	% wholesome	% wholesome	% pods bored	% seeds bored	% wholesome	% wholesome
(NO)	by *H. armigera*	by *H. armigera*	pods	seeds	by *H. armigera*	by *H. armigera*	pods	seeds	by *H. armigera*	by *H. armigera*	pods	seeds
Once in 3 wks	12.00	4.87	19.20	17.40	33.30	2.80	28.80	28.10	2,60	0.00	68.13	40.70
LSD 0.05	2.85	N.S	9.99	6.38	5.17	N.S	6.88	9.34	0.79	N.S	3.99	5.36
interaction												
(NO × F.)	N.S	N.S	N.S	14.26	N.S	N.S	N.S	N.S	N.S	N.S	N.S	N.S

Adopted from Dialoke, 2017.

The Use of Neem Seed Oil as an Alternative Insecticide for Grain Storage and Fruits/Vegetables Post Harvest Losses

Due to growing awareness of environmental issues and health hazards from synthetic pesticides, researchers now focus their attention on natural or otherwise called organic pesticides for grain storage purposes. Several plant materials have been exploited in protection of food commodities from insect infestations. Plant derived products namely, the azadirachtin from neem (*Azadirachta indica*), the pyrethrin from pyrethrum (*Chrysanthemum cinerariaefolium*), the carvone from caraway (*Carum carvi*) and the allyl isothiocynate from mustard (*Brassica nigra*) and horseradish (*Armoracia Rusticana*) oil have received global attention due to their pesticidal properties and potentials to protect several food commodities (Hartmans, et al. (1995; Ward, et al. 1998); Varma, et al. 1999; Athanassiou, et al.2005). The Neem seed oil can be used preventively as well as curatively. Thus, Bhatnagar et al. (2001), used different plant oils such as groundnut, sesame, soybean, coconut, mustard and neem oil at 10 ml/kg grain of grain and reported that the neem oil is the most effective against the pulse beetle *Callosobruchus maculatus* followed by coconut, soybean and mustard oil.

This traditional Indian tree which produces the Neem seed oil is also a good insect pest protectant. The toxicity of the Neem oil against the pulse beetle *Callosobruchus spp.* was studied in pulse grains and the persistent toxicity of the Neem oil was reported by Joana et al.(2010). Das, (1986), has reported percentage mortality within 4 days of release of pulse beetle in chickpea treated with 1% of neem oil. The Neem seed oil of 1% w/w and soft stone 0.5, 1.0% w/w and the neem seed kernel powder 4% w/w have been reported as grain protectant of pigeonpea against the pulse beetle *Callosobruchus chinensis* (Linn) (Singhal et al.1998). They also reported that the Neem seed kernel powder and the Neem seed oil protected the grains for a period of 8 months.

Table 10. Interaction of oil types and various concentrations of the oils on number of eggs laid by C. maculatus on cowpea samples after different storage periods

	Oil Concentrations (mL)						
Oil type	0	0.5	1	1.5	Mean	LSD at 0.05	Prob.of F.
		30 Days					
PN	686	10	23	10			
PM	283	105	25	15			
NM 1:1	891	37	66	26			
NM 1:2	955	34	34	22			
NM 1:3	649	34	27	26	190.90	185.8	<0.001
		60 Days					
PN	3667	10	20	8			
PM	2401	1474	247	15			
NM 1:1	3787	55	80	47			
NM 1:2	5073	38	36	33			
NM 1:3	5387	32	34	15	1123.00	1135.7	<0.001
		90 Days					
PN	6513	8	19	8			
PM	1163	1986	29	12			
NM 1:1	5607	64	63	45			
NM 1:2	3004	51	57	40			
NM 1:3	2862	36	30	21	1135.90	1275.5	<0.001
		120 Days					
PN	0	11	32	16			
PM	0	2137	1078	16			
NM 1:1	0	77	67	42			
NM 1:2	0	48	39	46			
NM 1:3	0	34	33	25	185.05	491.2	<0.001
		150 Days					
PN	0	14	20	8			
PM	0	2364	1737	18			
NM 1:1	0	88	62	38			
NM 1:2	0	38	50	39			
NM 1:3	0	36	31	22	228.50	338	<0.001
		180 Days					
PN	0	9.7	16	12			
PM	0	248	123.3	7.7			
NM 1:1	0	55.3	70.7	45.7			
NM 1:2	0	42.7	53.7	45.3			
NM 1:3	0	29	29.3	22	40.54	61.94	<0.001

Adopted from Singh et al. (2012).PN=Pure neem oil; PM=pure moringa; NM 1 : 1=neem-moringa oil in ratio 1 : 1; NM 1 : 2=neem-moringa oil in ratio 1 : 2; NM 1 : 3=neem-moringa oil in ratio 1 : 3.

A considerable amount of work has been carried out all over the world on the effect of plant extracts on the quality and shelf life in various fruit and vegetable crops. Fungal infections are one of the major causes of post harvest rots of fresh fruits and vegetables whether on transit or during storage. They cause significant economic losses in the commercialization phase, and are rendered unfit for human consumption (Anjum, et al., 2016).

The Neem oil may also kill the insect eggs. When the egg is already present at the surface of the seed or inside the seed, the oil coating prevents gaseous exchanges. So the larvae inside the egg or the kernel will die due to lack of oxygen. Some oils such as those derived from neem, karanja (*Pongamia glabra*), undi (*Calophyllum inophyllum*) and kusum (*Schleichera triguga*) also have an insecticidal effect, and a small amount may kill about 90% of the Cowpea weevil (*Callosobruchus maculatus*) (Singh et al. 2012). The protective effect may last for up to 3 months. There was no significant difference ($p>0.05$) in the activities of the oils in the first two months, but it indicated significant difference ($P<0.05$) in the third month between the oil types with the least number of eggs obtained from neen-moringa oil blend in the ratio of 1 : 3 and neem moringa oil in ratio 1 : 2 (737 and 788 eggs, resp.) (Table 10, Joana, et al., 2010). Pure Neem oil had the highest number of eggs (1637) at the third month. There was a sharp reduction in oviposition by *Callosobrucus maculatus* within the remaining three months for all the oil types except for pure moringa oil-treated samples that had the highest mean number (>800) of oviposition.

The pure Neem oil however appeared to be the best in reducing oviposition especially within the last three months of storage with less than 16 eggs laid, while pure moringa oil was the least with up to 1030 eggs in the fifth months of storage (Joana, et al., 2010). Rameshwar et al. (1987) observed that a combination of the neem leaf extract at 20% + UV radiation exposure for 10 minutes + rice starch 6% proved to be the most appropriate treatment in minimizing the reduction of juice contents and fruit rotting and fluctuation in physiological loss in weight was also minimum as compared to control. Wijewardane and Guleria (2009) studied about the concentration (1.5-2%) of neem oil as a surface coating along with pre-cooling at which 10°C was the most effective in providing a better physico-chemical umbrella, significantly lowering the fruit spoilage. The Neem oil surface coating along with shrink-wrapped tray packing at 2°C (85% to 90% RH) resulted in the longest storage life up to 150 days. Arya (1988) reported that higher concentration (75%) of leaf extract of the Neem was effective in reducing spores (82.3%) of two fruit rot pathogens, *Phomopsis psidii* and *Phomopsis viticola.* Sarvamangla (1993) studied the effect of leaf extracts from *Azadirachta indica*, *Calotropis gigantean*, *Calthranthus* sp. *Eucalyptus* sp., *Parthenium chysterophorus* and *Pongamia pinnata* on fruit quality of mulberry and reported that among these extracts the *Azadirachta indica* was the most effective in retaining higher sugar content, maintaining fruit size and shape, and resistance to fungal pathogens. The *Azadirachta indica* controlled the fungal pathogen more effectively as well as retaining the maximum sugar content as compare to *Calotropis gigantean*, *Calthranthus* spp. *Eucalyptus* spp., *Parthenium chysterophorus* and *Pongamia pinnata* ((Anjum, et al., 2016). Srivastava and Lal, (1997) reported that the leaf extract of the *Azadirachta indica* was effective in the control of fruit rot of pear and pomegranate. Deshmukh et al. (1992) have reported beneficial effects of Melia (*Melia Azadirachta*) and bavistin in controlling the storage fungi and insect-pests. They have also advocated the commercial use of Melia extract as a substitute for fungicides and insecticides.

CONCLUSION AND RECOMMENDATIONS

On a daily basis, farmers and the general public are exposed to toxic chemicals through the indiscriminate use of synthetic pesticides. Consequently, this research has highlighted the production, use and benefits of the Neem seed oil which is a botanical pesticide obtained from the Neem tree. The research further showed that the use of the Neem seed oil and the Neem cake provide an alternative and safe plant derived pesticides which serve as good substitute to synthetic pesticides. The uses of these botanical pesticides are beneficial in the effective control of pests as well as protection of the farmers' farmlands, soil, water and environment from the toxicity of the chemical pesticides. From the researches carried out on the use of the Neem seed oil, in Nigeria it was gathered that the weekly application of higher dosage of the Neem seed oil (6ml/litre of water equivalent to 12.5 ℓ in 840 litres of water ha^{-1}) at four weekly spraying regime controlled the population of okra beetles, plant vectors e.g., thrips podsucking bugs, podborers, and other pests infesting pigeonpea, okra, soybean crops etc. in farmers field. This rate also gave the best protection to the pigeonpea pods and seeds against damage especially when early maturing pigeonpea is planted and sprayed with formulated Neem seed oil (F-NSO) in July.

The Neem seed oil has been adjudged effective in the management of *R. dentipes,* thrips, *H. armigera*, etc., damage to pods and seeds, although it is less effective compared with the synthetic pyrethroid. However, because of the problems to human and environment associated with the use of these synthetic chemicals, the use of the formulated Neem seed oil is advocated. It is safe, economical and effective. In view of the efficacy, economical and safe use of the Neem seed oil, this research recommends it should be incorporated into the Integrated Pest Management (IPM) strategy in the rain forest environment of Owerri in Imo Stae, Nigeria.

Although, there are several limitations as earlier mentioned on the use of the neem seed oil to combat insect problems, however, to overcome these limitations, nanotechnology has emerged as a novel tool to address the problems of agricultural sustainability and food security (Khot et al. ,2012; kah and Hofmann, 2014, Kookana et al., 2014; Kal, 2015; Kashyap et al., 2015; Fraceto et al., 2016) Many studies have shown that the encapsulation of agrochemicals in nanoparticulate systems can enhance the efficacy of the active ingredient, decrease toxicity toward the environment and humans, and reduce losses due to volatilization, leaching, and photobleaching (Kulkami et al. 1999; Rivajan and Sakdapipanich, 2009; Devi and Maji, 2010; de Oliveira et al. 2014; Bakry et al., 2016; Gion et al., 2016).

From the point of view of sustainable agriculture, nanotechnology can help in the development of environmental friendly agricultural inputs, the improvement of the safety and stability of active agents, enhancement of their activity in pest control, and, consequently, increasing their acceptance by producers (Nair et al.2010; Srilatha, 2011; Khot et al., 2012; Agrawal and Rathore, 2014; Ram et al. 2014). The use of nanoparticles provides an effective means of protecting the neem oil against premature degradation, resulting in prolonging its effect on the target pest. The sustained release of the active agent is achieved, and environmental damage is minimal because the polymers employed are biodegradable. Furthermore, the number of applications of neem oil can be reduced, bringing substantial economic benefits (Kulkami et al. 1999; Isman et al.2001; Isman, 2006; de Oliveira et al., 2014; Isman and Grieneisen, 2014, Miresmailli and Isman, 2014). Although, the nanoencapsulation of neem oil has demonstrated good effects on insect pests, yet some issues need to be resolved so that the synergistic effect of nanoparticles associated with this botanical insecticide can significantly contribute to the control of insect pests. These issues include the need for: (1) A regulation of the use of nanomaterials in agriculture (2) Nanoformulations that are easily scalable (3) Comparative studies employing neem formulations available commercially to prove the cost/benefit of the nanoformulations; (4) A detailed studies of the degradation and behavior of these nanopesticides in the environment (5) An evaluation of toxicity towards non-target organisms (Joint Research Centre, 2015; Servin and White, 2015).

Due to the importance of the neem oil and its worldwide use for combating numerous pests in different crops, the nanoencapsulation of this oil should enable the production of more stable formulations for the control of insects that damage crops, especially those that are essential for human consumption. More so, the development of resistance in insects due to the indiscriminate use of neem oil to control pests would be solved by the use of nanotechnology.

This research also advocates that further studies be carried out to ascertain the practical application of the neem seed oil to solving grain storage and post harvest problems through Nanotechnology.

REFERENCES

Abdel-Shafy, S., and Zayed, A. A. (2002). "In vitro acaricidal effect of plant extract of neem seed oil (*Azadirachta indica*) on egg, immature, and adult stages of *Hyalomma anatolicum* excavatum (Ixodoidea: Ixodidae)." *Vet. Parasitol* 106 89–96.

Akhtar, M. (2000). "Nematicidal Potential of the neem tree *Azadirachta indica* (A. Juss)." *Journal of Integrated Pest Management Reviews* v. 5, n. 1, p. 57-66,

Agrawal, S., and Rathore, P. (2014). "Nanotechnology pros and cons to agriculture: a review." *Int. J.Curr. Microbiol. Appl. Sci*3:43–55.

Ahmad S., Ansari, M. S., and Muslim, M. (2015). "Toxic effects of neem based insecticides on the fitness of *Helicoverpa armigera* (Hübner)." *Crop Prot.*68:72–78.

Al-dabel, F., Mensih, R.K. and Frerot, B. (2007). The effects of nC24 and nC27 peroleum spray oils on oviposition and egg survival of *Ostrinia nubilalis* Hubner (Lepidoptera: Pyralidae) and *Trighogramma brassica* Bezdenko, adults on maize plants." *International Journal of pest management*;(In press).

Andresen, M. and Cedergreen, N. (2010)."Plant growth is stimulated by tea-seed extract: A new natural growth regulator?" *Hort Science* 45: 1848-1853.

Anjum, M. A., Ahmed, N., Chauhan, H., and Gupta, P. (2016). "Plant Extracts in Post-Harvest Disease Management of Fruits and Vegetables-A Review." *J Food Process Technol* 7:592.

Ansari, M.A., Mittal, P.K., Razdan, R.K., and Sreehari, U. (2005). "Larvicidal and mosquito repellent activities of Pine (*Pinus longifolia*, family: Pinaceae) oil." *J Vector Borne Dis*42:95–99.

Anuradha and Annadurai, R. S. (2008). "Biochemical and molecular evidence of azadirachtin binding to insect actins," *Current Science* vol. 95, no. 11, pp. 1588–1593.

Arya, A. (1988). "Control of phomosis fruit rot by leaf extract of certain medicinal plants." In: Kaushik P (eds.). *Indigenous Medicinal Plants.*

Symposium. Today and Tomorrows Printers and Publishers, New Delhi, 41-46.

Athanassiou, C.G., and Kavallieratos, N.G. (2005). Insecticidal effect and adherence of PyriSec in different grain commodities. *Crop Prot* 24: 703-710.

Bakry, A. M., Abbas, S., Ali B., Majeed, H., Abouelwafa, M. Y., and Mousa A., et al. (2016). "Microencapsulation of oils: a comprehensive review of benefits, techniques, and applications: encapsulation of marine, vegetable, essential oils." *Compr. Rev. Food Sci. Food Saf* 15:143–182.

Barnard, D.R., and Xue R.D. (2004). "Laboratory evaluation of mosquito repellents against *Aedes albopictus*, *Culex nigripalpus*, and *Ochierotatus triseriatus"* (Diptera: Culicidae) *J Med Entomol.* 41:726–730.

Basedow, T., Obiewatsch, H. R., Bernal Vega, J. A., Kollmann, S., and Nicol, C.M.Y. (2002). "Control of aphids and whiteflies Homoptera, Aphididae and Aleyrodidae) with different neem preparations in laboratory, greenhouse and field. Effects and limitations." *J. Plant Dis. Prot. 109: 612-623.*

Bhambal, A., Sonal, K., Saxena, S. and Manish, J. (2011). "Comparative effect of neem stick and toothbrush on plague removal and gingival heath- A clinical trial." *Journal of Advanced Oral Research* 2 (3): 51-56. ISSN 2229-4120.

Bhatnagar, A., Bhadauria, N. S. and Jakhmola, S.S. (2001). The efficacy of vegetable oils against pulse beetles Callosobruchus maculatus in cowpea. *Indian J.Entomol*. 63:237-239.

Blaney, W.M., Sommonds, M.S.J., Ley, W.V., Anderson, J.C. and Toogood, P.L. (1990). "Antifeedant effects of azadirachtin and structurally related compounds on lepidopterous larvae." *Entomol. Exp. Appl* 55:149-160.

Bilton, J.N., Broughton, H.B., Jones, P.S., Ley, S.V., Lidert, Z., Morgan, E.D., Rzepa, H.S., Sheppard, R.N., Slawin, A.M.Z. and Williams D.J.(1987). "An X-ray crystallographic, mass spectroscopic, and NMR study of the limonoid insect antifeedant azadirachtin and related derivatives." *Tetrahedron* 43: 2805-2815.

Boeke, S. J., Boersma, M. G., Alink, G. M., van Loon, J. J., van Huis, A., and Dicke, M., et al. (2004). "Safety evaluation of neem (*Azadirachta indica*) derived pesticides." *J. Ethnopharmacol* 94:25–41.

Brahmachari,G.(2004). "Neem–an omnipotent plant: a retrospection." *Chembiochem* 5:408–421.

Butterworth, J.H. and Morgan, E.D. (1968)."Isolation of a substance that suppresses feeding in locusts." *J. Chem. Soc., Chem. Commun.* 23-24.

Callahan, C. (2010). *Uses of Neem Datun for Teeth,* Livestrong.com Demand Media https://en.wikipedia.org/wiki/*Azadirachta_indica.*

Caraballo, A.J. 2000. "Mosquito repellent action of Neemos." *J Am Mosq Control Assoc* 16:45–46.

Chi, Y.C., Sakamaki, C.Y., and Kushigema, K. (2003). "The seasonal abundance of podborer, *Maruca vitrata* in Kagoshima, Japan." *Members of the Faculty of Agriculture, Kagoshima University* 35: 41-44.

Cox, C. (2002). "Pyrethrins/pyrethrum insecticide factsheet." *J. Pestic. Reform*22:14–20.

Das, G.P. (1986). "Persisitant toxicity of neem oil against the pulse beetle *Callosobruchus chinensis* Linn. in different pulse grains. " *Bangladesh J Zool* 14:15-18.

Degri, M.M., and Hadi, H.M.,(2000). "Field evaluation and economies of some insecticides against the major pests of cowpea (*Vigna unguiculata* (L.) Walp, in Bauchi, Nigeria." *ESN occasional publication 32:113-118.*

Deshmukh, P.B., Chavam, S.R., and Rehapukar, D.M. (1992). "A study of insecticidal activity of twenty indigenous plants." *Pesticide* 16:7-10.

Desai, M. V. et al. (1979). "Oil-cakes in control of root-not nematodes." *Tobacco Research* 5:105-108.

Dialoke, S.A., Agu, C.M., Ojiako, F.O, Onweremadu, E., Onyishi, G.O., Ozor, N., Echezona, B.C.,Ofor, M.O., Ibeawuchi, I.I., Chigbundu, I.N., Ngwuta, A.A., and Ugwoke, F.O. (2010). "Survey of insect pests on pigeon pea in Nigeria." *Journal of SAT Agricultural Research 8*:1-8.

Dialoke, S.A., Emosairue, S.O., Egho, E.O., and Ogoke, I.J.(2014a). "Insect species associated with early maturing pigeon pea in Nigeria." *Indian Journal of Entomology* 76(4): 330-336ISSN: 0367-8288.

Dialoke, S.A., Ogoke, I. J., Ngwuta, A.A., and Ofor, M.O. (2014b). "Sustainable production of improved pigeonpea pods through management of *Riptortus dentipes* Fab. (Hemiptera: coreidae) with formulated neem seed oil at varying rates and spraying schedules in Owerri, Nigeria." *Indian Journal of biopesticides* 7 (1): 85-89.

Dialoke, S.A., Bosah, O.A., and Uluocha, O.B. (2014c). The "Efficacy of different rates of formulated neem seed oil and frequency of application on the control of flower thrips infesting early maturing pigeonpea cultivar in Owerri, Imo State, Nigeria." *Journal of Natural Science Research* Vol.4:22:61-65.

Dialoke, S.A., Ngwuta, A.A., Ofor, M.O., Uluocha, O.B., and Nwokeji,E.M. (2015a). The "Efficacy of neem oils in the management of okra flea beetle (*Podagrica* spp), in the rainforest, zone of South Eastern, Nigeria." *Journal of Biopesticides and Environment* 1:42-49.

Dialoke, S.A., Ojiako, F.O. and Nwokeji, E. M. (2015b). Effect of formulated neem seed oil (F-NSO) at different rates and frequencies on the population of short duration pigeon-pea flower beetle (*Aulacophora vinula* Eric) in Owerri rainforest Zone, Nigeria.

Dialoke, S.A. (2017). Effect of Neem Seed Oil on *Helicoverpa armigera* on pigeonpea in Nigeria. *Indian Journal of Entomology*, 7 (2): 125-129.

de Oliveira J. L., Campos, E. V. R., Bakshi, M., Abhilash, P. C., and Fraceto, L. F. (2014). "Application of nanotechnology for the encapsulation of botanical insecticides for sustainable agriculture: prospects and promises." *Biotechnol. Adv.* 32:1550–1561.

Devi, N., and Maji, T. K. (2010). "Genipin crosslinked microcapsules of gelatin A and κ-carrageenan polyelectrolyte complex for encapsulation of Neem (*Azadirachta Indica* A. Juss.) seed oil." *Polym. Bull.* 65:347–362.

Dremova, V.P., Markina, V.V., and Kamennov, N.A. (1971). "How evaporation and absorption affect the formulation of various insect repellents." *Int Pest Cont* 13:13–16.

Drew, R.A. (1992). "Clonal propagation of *Azadirachta indica* and field testing of *Azadirachtin* in some vegetable crops," *Final Report for RIRDC Project*No DAQ 59A

Dubey, N. K., Shukla R., Kumar A., Singh P., and Prakash B. (2010). "Prospects of botanical pesticides in Sustainable Agriculture." *Curr. Sci.*98:479–480.

Emosairue, S.O., and Ubana, U.B. (1996). "Field evaluation of neem for the control of some insect pests in south East Nigeria." *Journal of Applied chemistry and Agricultural Research* 4:237-241.

Emosairue, S.O., and Ukeh, D.A. (1996). "Field trial of neem production for the control of okra flea beetle (*Podagrica* spp.) in Southeastern Nigeria." *African Journal for Plant Protection* 6:22-26.

Emosairue, S.O. (2007). "Nature of damage of Insect to crops." In: *Fundamentals of Agricultural Entomology, for use in tertiary schools and institutions*, Ethiope Publishing Corporation, Ring Road Benin City, Nig, 91-213. ISBN 978-123-083.

Esmaeili, A., and Asgari, A. (2015). "In vitro release and biological activities of *Carum copticum* essential oil (CEO) loaded chitosan nanoparticles." *Int. J. Biol. Macromol* 81:283–290.

Estefania, V. R.C., Jhones, L. O., Monica, P., Renata, L. and Leonard, F.F. (2016). "Neem Oil and Crop Protection: From Now to the Future." *Online Front Plant Sci* 7:1494.

FAO, (1988). "Traditional food plants." *Food and Agricultural Organisation of the United Nations*, Rome.

Feng, R., and Isman, M. B. (1995). "Selection for resistance to azadirachtin in the green peach aphid" *Myzus persicae.Experientia* 51:831–833. 10.1007/BF01922438.

Fraceto, L. F., Grillo, R., de Medeiros, G. A., Scognamiglio, V., Rea, G., and Bartolucci, C. (2016). "Nanotechnology in agriculture: which innovation potential does it have?" *Front. Environ. Sci* 4:20.

Gahukar, R. T. (2014). "Factors affecting content and bioefficacy of neem (*Azadirachta indica* A. Juss.) phytochemicals used in agricultural pest control: a review." *Crop Prot* 62:93–99.

Garg, S.C. and Siddiqui, N. 1992. "Antifungal activity of some essential oils isolates." *Pharmazie* 47:467-468.

Ghosh, A., Chowdhury, N., and Chandra, G. (2012). "Plant extracts as potential mosquito larvicides."*Indian J. Med. Res* 135:581–598.

Giongo, A. M. M., Vendramim, J. D., and Forim, M. R. (2016). "Evaluation of neem-based nanoformulations as alternative to control fall armyworm." *Ciênc. Agrotec* 40:26–36.

Girish, K., and Shankara Bhat, S. (2008). 'Neem–a green treasure." *Electron. J. Biol.* 4:102–111.

Gonzalez-Coloma, A., Reina, M., Diaz, C. E., Fraga, B. M., and Santana-Meridas O. (2013). "Natural product-based biopesticides for insect control," in *Reference Module in Chemistry, Molecular Sciences and Chemical Engineering* ed. Reedijk J., editor. (Amsterdam: Elsevier).

Guillette, J. (1994). "Development of abnormalities of the gonad and abnormal sex hormone concentration in juvenile alligators from contaminated and control lakes in Environ." *Health Perspect, Florida vol.102:680-688.*

Gopali, J.B., Teggelli, R., Mannur, D.M. and Yelshetty, S. (2010). Web forming lepidopteran, *Maruca vitrata* Geyer. "An emerging and destructive pest of pigeonpea." *Karnataka J. Agric. Sci.* 23(1):35-38.

Hartmans, K.J., Diepenhorst, P., Bakker, W., and Gorris, L.G.M. (1995). The use of carvone in agriculture, sprout suppression of potatoes and antifungal activity against potato tuber and other plant diseases. *Ind Crop Prod* 4: 3-13.

Hasan F., and Shafiq Ansari, M. (2011). "Toxic effects of neem-based insecticides on *Pieris brassicae* (Linn.)." *Crop Prot* 30:502–507.

Henrick, C.A. (1995). "Pyrethroid." In *Agrochemicals from natural products,* edited by Godfrey, C.R.A. New York, Basil, Hong Kong, Marcel Dekker, Inc., 63-145

Isman, M. B. (2006). "Botanical Insecticides, Deterrents, and Repellents in Modern Agriculture and an Increasingly Regulated World." *Annu. Rev. Entomol.*51:45–66.

Isman, M. B., Wan, A. J., and Passreiter, C. M. (2001). "Insecticidal activity of essential oils to the tobacco cutworm, *Spodoptera litura*." *Fitoterapia* 72:65–68.

IITA. (1993). *International Institutes of Tropical Agriculture Research*, No.7: 5-8.

Jackai, L. E. N., and Oyediran, O. A. (1991). "The potential of neem, Azadirachta indica for controlling post flowering pests of cowpea, *Vigna unguiculata* (l.) Walp. 1: The pod borer, *Maruca testulalis*." *Geyer, Insect Sci. Appl c* 12 (1/2/3/): 103-109.

Jackai, L.E.N., (1993). "The use of neem in controlling cowpea pests." *ITTA Research No.7.*

Jackai, L.E.N. and Adalla, C.B. (1997). "Pest management practices in cowpea." A Review." In *Advances in Cowpea Research* (Dashiel, K.E., D. R. Mohan Raju and B.B. Singh Eds.) Sayce Publishing Devon U.K., 240-258.

Joana, O. Ilesanmi I, and Daniel, T. (2010). "Preservation of Cowpea (Vigna unguiculata (L.) Walp) Grains against Cowpea Bruchids (Callosobruchus maculatus) Using Neem and Moringa Seed Oils." *International Journal of Agronomy* Volume 1-8.

Joint Research Centre (2015). "*Nano in Food and Agriculture: Regulations Require Collaboration to Ensure Safety – EU Science Hub – European Commission. EU Science Hub.*" Accessed June 16, 2016. Available at: https://ec.europa.eu/jrc/en/news/nano-food-and-agriculture-regulations-require-collaboration-ensure-safety].

Kah, M. (2015). "Nanopesticides and nanofertilizers: emerging contaminants or opportunities for risk mitigation?" *Front. Chem.* 3:64.

Kah, M., and Hofmann, T. (2014). "Nanopesticide research: current trends and future priorities." *Environ. Int.* 63:224–235.

Karungi, J., Adipala, E., Ogenga-latigo, M.W., Kyamanywa, S., and Oyobo, N., (2000). "Pest management in cowpea. Part 1: Influence of planting time and plant density on cowpea field pests infestation in Eastern, Uganda." *Crop protection* 19:231-136.

Kashyap, P. L., Xiang, X., and Heiden, P. (2015). "Chitosan nanoparticle based delivery systems for sustainable agriculture." *Int. J. Biol. Macromol* 77:36–51.

Khan, A. M.; Alam, M. M. and Ahmad, R. (1974). "Mechanisms of control of plant parasitic nematodes as a result of the application of oil-cakes to the soil." *Indian Journal of Nematology*4:93-96.

Khot, L. R., Sankaran, S., Maja, J. M., Ehsani, R., and Schuster, E. W. (2012). "Applications of nanomaterials in agricultural production and crop protection: a review." *Crop Prot*35:64–70.

Khurana, A.D. (1997). "Seasonal activity and chemical control of *Helicoverpaarmigera* Hubner on chickpea." *J. Insect Sci* 10: 48-51

Kimani, P.M., (1987). "Pigeonpea breeding in Kenya." Objectives and Methods, In: *Proceedings of pigeonpea scientists meet*, 2-5, Jun. 1987, Nairobi, Kenya. Patancheru, A.P. 502 324, India, ICRISAT.

Kogan, M. (1998). "Integrated pest management: historical perspectives and contemporary developments." *Annu. Rev. Entomol* 43:243–270.

Kookana, R. S., Boxall, A. B. A., Reeves, P. T., Ashauer, R., Beulke, S., and Chaudhry, Q. et al. (2014). "Nanopesticides: guiding principles for regulatory evaluation of environmental risks." *J. Agric. Food Chem*62:4227–4240.

Koul, O., Isman, M. B. and Ketkar, C. M. (1990). "Properties and uses of neem, Azadirachta indica." *Canadian Journal of Botany*, v. 68, 1:1-11.

Koul, O. and Isman M.B. (1991). "Effects of azadirachtin on the dietary utilization and development of the variegated cutworm *Peridroma saucia*." *J. Insect. Physiol* 37:591-598.

Kraus, W., Bokel, M. Bruhn, A. Cramer, R. Klaiber, I. Klenck, A., Nagl, G., Pöhnl, H., Sadlo, H. and Vogler, B.(1987). "Structure determination by NMR of azadirachtin and related compounds from *Azadirachta indica* (Meliaceae)." *Tetrahedron* 43:2817-2830.

Kulkarni, A. R., Soppimath, K. S., Aminabhavi, T. M., Dave, A. M., and Mehta, M. H. (1999). "Urea–formaldehyde crosslinked starch and guar gum matrices for encapsulation of natural liquid pesticide [*Azadirachta*

Indica A. Juss. (neem) seed oil]: swelling and release kinetics." *J. Appl. Polym. Sci*73:2437–2446.

Kwon, Y., Kim, S.H., Ronderos, D.S., Lee, Y., Akitake, B., Woodward, O.M., Guggino, W.B., Smith, D.P., and Montell, C. (2010). "Drosophila TRPA1 channel is required to avoid the naturally occurring insect repellent citronellal." *Curr Biol* 20:1672–1678.

Kyamanywa, S., Akonga, T., and Rubaihayo, P.R., (2001). "Past and current studies on ecology and management of insect pests of pigeonpea." In: Silim, S.N., Mergeai, G., and Kimani, P.M., (eds.) (2000). *Status and potential of pigeonpea in Eastern and Southern Africa;* Proceedings of a Regional Legume workshop 12-15 September 2000, Nairobi Kenya. ICRISAT.

Liao, C.T. and Lin, C.S. (2000). "Occurrence of the legume podborer, *Maruca testulalis* Geyer (Lepidoptera: Pyralidae) on cowpea (*Vigna unguiculata* Walp) and its insecticides application trial." *Plant prot. Bull. Taipei* 42 (4):213-222.

Locke, J. (1994). "Neem Oil Locks out Spores." *Agricultural Research*.

Lokanadhan, S., Muthukrishnan, P., and Jeyaraman S. 2012. "Neem products and their agricultural applications." *J. Biopestic* 5:72–76.

Lucantoni, L., Giusti, F., Cristofaro, M., Pasqualini, L., Esposito, F., and Lupetti, P., et al. (2006). "Effects of a neem extract on blood feeding, oviposition and oocyte ultrastructure in *Anopheles stephensi* Liston (Diptera: Culicidae)." *Tissue Cell* 38:361–371.

Mancebo, F., Hilje, L., Mora, G. A., and Salazar, R. (2002). "Biological activity of two neem (*Azadirachta indica* A. Juss., Meliaceae) products on *Hypsipyla grandella* (Lepidoptera: Pyralidae) larvae." *Crop Prot* 21:107–112.

Manjunath, T.M., Bhatnagar, V.S., Pawar, C.S., and Sithanantham, S. (1995). *"Economic importance of Heliothis spp. In India and assessment of their natural enemies and host plants"*. Paper presented for the international workshop on Biological control of Heliothis spp. 11-15 November, New Delhi, India.

Marco, M.P., Pascal, N., Bellies, X., Camps, S., and Messeguer, A., (1990). "Ecdysteroid depletion by *Azadirachtin* in *Tenebrio monitor* pupae." *Pesticide Biochemistry and physiology* 38:60-65.

Mathur S., and Kachhwaha, S. (2015). Neem tree: amazing beauty component in skin and hair care.*Adv. Pharmacol. Toxicol.*16 31–43.

Mayilswami, S. and Reid, B. (2010). "Effect of earthworms on nutrients dynamics in soil and growth of crop." *Research Journal of Chemistry and Environment* v. 14, n. 2, 39-44.

Michereff-Filho, M., Torres, J. B., Andrade, L. N., and Nunes, M. U. C. (2008). "Effect of some biorational insecticides on Spodoptera eridania in organic cabbage." *Pest Manag. Sci.*64:761–767.

Miresmailli, S., and Isman, M. B. (2014). "Botanical insecticides inspired by plant–herbivore chemical interactions." *Trends Plant Sci.*19:29–35.

Mohanty, S., Patra, A., and Chhonkar, P. (2008). "Neem (*Azadirachta indica*) seed kernel powder retards urease and nitrification activities in different soils at contrasting moisture and temperature regimes." *Bioresour. Technol.*99:894–899.

Moore, S. J,, Lenglet, A., and Hill, N. (2002). "Field evaluation of three plant-based insect repellents against malaria vectors in Vaca Diez Province, the Bolivian Amazon." *J Am Mosq Control Assoc*107–110.

Mordue, (Luntz), A.J., Cottee P.K. and Evans K.A. (1985). "Azadirachtin: Its effect on gut motility, growth and moulting in *locusta*." *Physiol. Entomol* 10:431-437.

Mordue, (Luntz) A. J., and Blackwell, A. (1993). "Azadirachtin: an update." *J. Insect Physiol.*39:903–924.

Mordue, (Luntz), A.J., Nisbet, A.J., Nasiruddin, M. and Walker, E. (1996). "Differential thresholds of azadirachtin for feeding deterrence and toxicity in locusts and an aphid". *Entomol. Exp. Appl* 80:69-72.

Mordue, (Luntz), A.J., Simmonds, M.S.J., Ley, S.V., Blaney, W. M., Mordue, W., Nasiruddin, M., and Nisbet A.J. (1998)."Actions of azadirachtin, a plant allelochemical, against insects." *Pestic. Sci.* 54:277-284.

Mordue, (Luntz), A.J., Nisbet, A.J., Jennens, L., Ley, S.V., and Mordue, W. (1999). Tritated hihydroazadirachtin binding to *Schistocerca gregaria* testes and Spodoptera Sf9 cells suggests a similar cellular mechanism of action for azadirachtin." In R.P. Singh & R.C. Saxena (eds.), *Azadirachta indica*, A. 247-258. Juss. Int. Neem Conference, Gatton, Australia 1996. Oxford & IBH Publ. Co. PVT Ltd.

Mordue, A. J. and Nisbet, A. J. (2000). "Azadirachtin from the neem tree Azadirachta indica: its action against insects," *Anais da Sociedade Entomologica do Brazil*, vol. 29 (4): 615–632. *Print version* ISSN 0301-8059 On-line version ISSN 1981-5328.

Morgan, E. D. (2009). "Azadirachtin, a scientific gold mine." *Bioorg. Med. Chem.*17:4096–4105.

Muangphra, P., and Gooneratne, R., (2011). "Toxicity of Commercial Neem Extract to Earthworms (Pheretima peguana)." *Applied and Environmental Soil Science v* 1–8.

Mulla, M. S., and Su, T. (1999). "Activity and biological effects of neem products against arthropods of medical and veterinary importance." *J. Am. Mosq. Control Assoc.*15:133–152.

Musalia, L., Anandan, S., Sastry, V. R., and Agrawal, D. (2000). "Urea-treated neem (*Azadirachta indica* A. juss) seed kernel cake as a protein supplement for lambs." *Small Rumin. Res.*35:107–116.

Naik, D. J., V. V. Belavadi, D. Thippesha, M. D. Kumar, and D. Madaiah, (2006)."Field efficacy of neem products against thrips and capsule borer of small soy bean," *Karnataka Journal of Agricultural Sciences*, vol. 19, no. 1, pp. 144–145, 2006.

Nair, R., Varghese, S. H., Nair, B. G., Maekawa, T., Yoshida, Y., and Kumar, D. S. (2010). "Nanoparticulate material delivery to plants." *Plant Sci.*179:154–163.

Nasiruddin, M. and Mordue, (Luntz) A.J. (1993). "The effect azadirachtin on the midgut histology of the locusts, *Schistocerca gregaria* and *Locusta migratoria*." *Tissue Cell* 25:875-884.

Nicoletti, M., Petitto, V., Gallo, F. R., Multari, G., Federici, E., and Palazzino, G. (2012). "The modern analytical determination of botanicals and similar novel natural products by the HPTLC fingerprint approach." *Stud. Nat. Prod. Chem* 37:217–258.

Night, G. and Ogenga-Latigo, M.W. (1994). "Range and occurrence of pigeonpea (*Cajanus cajan*) pests in Central Uganda." *African Crop Science Journal* 2 (1):105-109.

Ni, K., Pacholski, A., and Kage, H. (2014). "Ammonia volatilization after application of urea to winter wheat over 3 years affected by novel urease and nitrification inhibitors." *Agric. Ecosyst. Environ.*197:184–194.

Nisbet, A.J. (1992). "*The effect of azadirachtin on the feeding behaviour and virus transmission of Myzus persicae (Sulzer).*" PhD thesis, University of Glasgow, 312p.

Nisbet, A.J., Woodford, J.A.T. Strang R.H.C. and Connolly, J.D. (1993). "Systemic antifeedant effects of azadirachtin on the peach-potato aphid *Myzus persicae*." *Entomol. Exp. Appl* 68:87-98.

Nisbet, A.J., Woodford, J.A.T., and Strang R.H.C. (1994)."The effects of azadirachtin-treated diets on the feeding behaviour and fecundity of the peach-potato aphid, *Myzus persicae.*" *Entomol. Exp. Appl* 71:65-72.

Niu, J. Z., Hull-Sanders, H., Zhang, Y. X., Lin, J. Z., Dou, W., and Wang, J.J. (2014). "Biological control of arthropod pests in citrus orchards in China." *Biol. Control* 68:15–22.

Norten, E. and Pütz, J. (1999). "*Neem: India's Miraculous Healing Plant.*" Rochester, VT: Inner Traditions/Bear & Co.

NRC (National Research Council), (1992). *"A tree for solving global problems."* National Academy press, Washington D.C, 31-37.

Ogbuewu, I. P., Odoemenam, V. U., Obikaonu, H. O., Opara, M. N., Emenalom, O. O., and Uchegbu, M. C., et al. (2011). "The growing importance of neem (*Azadirachta indica* A. Juss) in agriculture, industry, medicine and environment: a review." *Res. J. Med. Plant* 5:230–245.

Olaifa, J.I., Adedokun, S.A., and Adenuga, A.D. (1991). "Anti-feedant and growth regulating effects of neem products on the variegated grass hopper (*Zonocerus variegatus* L.)" *Orthoptera: Pyromorphidae. J. African Zool* 105 (2):157-162.

Okunlola, A.I., and Ofuya, T.I. (2013). "Effect of mixed cropping and plant extracts on the growth, yield and pest control of jute (*Corchorusolitorius* L.)." *Folia Horticult* 25:49-60.

Oparaeke, A.M. (2005). "Effects of aqueous extracts of tropical plants for management of *Maruca vitrata* Fab. And *Clavigralla tomentosicollis* Stal. on cowpea, *Vigna unguiculata* (L.) Walp. plants." *Asian Journal of Entomology* 1:1-5.

Oparaeke, A.M., Dike, M.C., and Amatobi, C.I. (2006). "Insecticidal efficacy of SABRUKA formulations asprotectants of cowpea against field crops." *Journal of Entomology*1-6.

Pandey, A.K. (1980). "Effect of benzene hexachloride—insecticides on the testicular histology in *Tilapia mossambica*, *Geogios*, 7: 251-253.

Pant, M., Dubey, S., and Patanjali, P. K. (2016). "Recent advancements in bio-botanical pesticide formulation technology development." In*Herbal Insecticides, Repellents and Biomedicines: Effectiveness and Commercialization* eds. Veer, V., Gopalakrishnan, R., editors. (New Delhi: Springer), 117–126.

Pereira, J. (1983). Effectiveness of six vegetable oils protectants of cowpeas and bambara groundnut infestation by *Callosobruchus maculatus* in *Stored Products, Res.,* 19:59-62.

PMC (2011). "An overview of repellent neem oil efficacy from literature review." *Malar J.* 10(1):11

Qiao, J., Zou, X., Lai, D., Yan, Y., Wang, Q., and Li, W., et al. (2014). "Azadirachtin blocks the calcium channel and modulates the cholinergic miniature synaptic current in the central nervous system of *Drosophila*." *Pest Manag. Sci.*70:1041–1047.

Quarles, W. (1994). "Neem Tree Pesticides Protect Ornamental Plants." *The IPM Practitioner* 16(10):1-13.

Raheja, A.K. (1973). "Onion thrips and their control in Northern, Nigeria." *Samaru Agric. News.* 15(2):82-86.

Rajabaskar, D. and Regupathy, A. (2013). "Neem based IPM modules for control of Scirtothrips soybeans Rank and Conogethes punctiferalis Gunee in small soy bean," *Asian Journal of Biological Sciences,* vol. 6, no. 3, pp. 142–152.

Ram, P., Vivek, K., and Kumar, S. P. (2014). "Nanotechnology in sustainable agriculture: present concerns and future aspects." *Afr. J. Biotechnol.*13:705–713.

Rameshwar, Dayal, J., Ram, S, et al. (1987). Role of Post-harvest treatment with plant extracts, ultra violet radiation and rice starch on keeping quality of Sweet Orange (*Citrus sinesis osbeck*) cv. mosambi. *J Eco Physiol.*

Rehman, J. U., Ali, A., and Khan, I. A. (2014). "Plant based products: use and development as repellents against mosquitoes: a review." *Fitoterapia* 95:65–74.

Rekha, S. and Mallur, C.P. (2007). "Studies of insect pests of Dolichos bean in Northern Karnataka." *Karnataka J. Agric. Sci* 20(2):407-409.

Rembold, H and Annadurai, R. S. (1993). "Azadirachtin inhibits proliferation of Sf9 cells in monolayer culture." *Z. Naturforsch* 48:495-499.

Riyajan, S. A., and Sakdapipanich, J. T. (2009). "Encapsulated neem extract containing Azadiractin-A within hydrolyzed poly(vinyl acetate) for controlling its release and photodegradation stability." *Chem. Eng. J.*152:591–597.

Rouf, F. M. A. and Sardar, M. A. (2011). "Extract of crude seed extract of some indigenous plants for the control of legume pod borer (*Maruca vitrata*) on country bean." *Bangladesh J. Agril Res* 361:41-50.

Roychoudhury R. 2016. "Neem products," in *Ecofriendly Pest Management for Food Security* ed. Omkar, editor. (Amsterdam: Elsevier) 545–562.

Sahoo, B.K. (1995). "Extent of damage by web forming Lepidoptera pod borers on pigeonpea." *Indian J. pulses Res* 8:195-196.

Sakulku, U., Nuchuchua, O., Uawongyart, N., Puttipipatkhachorn, S., Soottitantawa, T.A., and Ruktanonchai, U. (2009). "Characterization and mosquito repellent activity of citronella oil nanoemulsion." *Int J Pharm*372:105–111.

Sarvamangla, H.S. (1993). "Evaluation of plant extract for the control of fungal disease of blackberry." *Indian Phytopath* 46:398-401.34.

Simmonds, M.S.J., Blaney, W.M., Ley, S.V., Anderson, J. C., and Toogood, P.L., (1990). "Azadirachtin: Structural requirements for reducing growth and increasing mortality in lepidopterous larvae." *Entomol. Exp. Appl* 55:169-181.

Schmutterer, H. (ed.) (1985). "The neem tree *Azadirachtia indica* A. Juss and other meliaceous plants: Sources of unique natural products for integrated pest management, medicine, industry and other purposes." *VCH, Weinheim, Germany* 696p.

Schmutterer, H. (1990). "Properties and potential of natural pesticides from the neem tree, Azadirachta indica." *Ann. Rev. Entomol* 35:271-298.

Schmutterer, H. and Singh, R.P. (1995). "List of insect Pests susceptible to neem products. In: Schmutterer, H. (Ed.)." *The Neem tree: Azadirachta indicaA. Juss and other Meliacious plants VCH, New York* 326-365. North America. Coleopterists Bulletin 57:369-381.

Schmutterer, H., and Singh, K. P., (2002). "List of insect Pests susceptible to neem products." In: Schmutterer, H. (Ed.). *The Neem tree: Azadirachtaindica A. Juss and other Meliacious plants-sources of Unique Natural Products for Integrated Pest Management, Medicine, Industry and other purposes.* 2nd Edn., Neem Foundation. Mumbai India, 411-456.

Scudeler, E. L., and dos Santos, D. C. (2013). "Effects of neem oil (*Azadirachta indica* A. Juss) on midgut cells of predatory larvae *Ceraeochrysa claveri* (Neuroptera: Chrysopidae)." *Micron.* 44:125–132.

Scudeler, E. L., Garcia, A. S. G., Padovani, C. R., and Santos, D. C. (2013). "Action of neem oil (*Azadirachta indica* A. Juss) on cocoon spinning in *Ceraeochrysa claveri* (Neuroptera: Chrysopidae)." *Ecotoxicol. Environ. Saf.* 97:176–182.

Scudeler, E. L., Padovani, C. R., and dos Santos, D. C. (2014). "Effects of neem oil (*Azadirachta indica* A. Juss) on the replacement of the midgut epithelium in the lacewing *Ceraeochrysa claveri* during larval-pupal metamorphosis." *Acta Histochem* 116:771–780.

Seljåsen, R., and Meadow, R. (2006). "Effects of neem on oviposition and egg and larval development of *Mamestra brassicae* L: dose response, residual activity, repellent effect and systemic activity in cabbage plants." *Crop Prot* 25:338–345.

Senguttuvan, T., and Rajendran, R. (2001). "Plant products for the control of bhendi fruit borers," in Proceedings of the 2nd National Symposium on Integrated Pest Management (IPM) in *Horticultural Crops: New Molecules, Biopesticides and Environment*, Bangalore, India 17–18,

Senthil Nathan, S., Choi, M. Y., Seo, H. Y., Paik, C. H., and Kalaivani, K. (2009). "Toxicity and behavioral effect of 3β,2425-trihydroxycycloartane and beddomei lactone on the rice leaffolder *Cnaphalocrocis medinalis* (Guenée) (Lepidoptera: Pyralidae)." *Ecotoxicol. Environ. Saf.* 72:1156–1162.

Senthil Nathan, S., Kalaivani, K., Sehoon, K., and Murugan, K. (2006). "The toxicity and behavioural effects of neem limonoids on *Cnaphalocrocis medinalis* (Guenée), the rice leaffolder." *Chemosphere* 62:1381–1387.

Servin, A. D., and White, J. C. (2016). "Nanotechnology in agriculture: next steps for understanding engineered nanoparticle exposure and risk."*Nanoimpact*1:9–12.

Shanower, T.G., Romeis, J. and Minja, E.M. (1999). "Insect pests of pigeonpea and management." *Ann. Rev. Ent.*, 44:77-96.

Sharma, V. P., Ansari, M. A., and Razdan, R.K. 1993. "Mosquito repellent action of neem *(Azadirachta indica)* oil." *J Am Mosq Control Assoc* 9:359–360.

Sheldarke, A.R., and Narayanan, N. (1979). "Pulse physiology." *Annual Report 1976, part Pigeonpea, Patancheru*, A.P. 502 324, India. ICRISAT (Semi-formal publications).

Seufert, V., Ramankutty, N., and Foley, J. A. (2012). "Comparing the yields of organic and conventional agriculture." *Nature* 485:229–232.

Siegwart, M., Graillot, B., Blachere Lopez, C., Besse, S., Bardin, M., and Nicot, P. C., et al. (2015). "Resistance to bio-insecticides or how to enhance their sustainability: a review." *Front. Plant Sci.* 6:381

Singhal, S.K., Chauhan, R., Dahiya, B. (1998). "Evaluation of some plant products and nontoxic materials for protection of pigeonpea against *Callososbruchus chinensis" Linn. J of Insect Sci* 11:181-183.

Singh, N., Mishra, A. K., and Saxena, A. (1996). "Use of neem cream as a mosquito repellent in tribal areas of central India." *Indian J Malariol*33:99–102.

Singh, A., Khare, A., and Singh, A. P., (2012). Use of Vegetable Oils as Biopesticide in Grain Protection -A Review." *J Biofertil Biopestici* 3:114.

Soundararajan, R. P. and Lakshmanan, V. (2009). "Neem in pest management of horticultural crops," In *Neem, A Treatise*, K. K. Singh, Ed., 546, I. K. International Pvt Ltd, New Delhi, India.

Srilatha, B. (2011). "Nanotechnology in agriculture." *J. Nanomed. Nanotechnol* 2:123.

Srivastava, A.K., and Lal, P. (1997). "Studies on bio fungicidal properties of leaf extracts of some plant." *Indian Phytopath* 50:408-411

Stanley, J.S. Chandrasekaran, G. Preetha, and Kuttalam, S., (2010). "Physical and biological compatibility of diafenthiuron with micro/macro nutrients fungicides and biocontrol agents used in soy bean," *Archives of Phytopathology and Plant Protection* vol. 43, no. 14, pp. 1396–1406.

Stone, R. (1992). "A Biopesticidal Tree Begins to Blossom." *Science*.

Sujarwo, W., Keim, A. P., Caneva, G., Toniolo, C., and Nicoletti, M. 2016. "Ethnobotanical uses of neem (*Azadirachta indica* A. Juss.; Meliaceae) leaves in Bali (Indonesia) and the Indian subcontinent in relation with historical background and phytochemical properties." *J. Ethnopharmacol* 189:186–193.

Syed, Z., and Leal, W.S. (2008). "Mosquitoes smell and avoid the insect repellent DEET." *Proc Natl Acad Sci U.S.A.* 10:1073.

Takahashi, S., Mukai, H., Tanabe, S., Sakayama, Miyazaki, T., and Musano, H. (1999). "Butyl tin residues in livers of humans and wild terrestrial mammals, and in plastics products." *Environmental pollution*106:213-218.

Tangtrakulwanich, K., and Reddy, G. V. P. (2014). "Development of insect resistance to plant biopesticides: an overview," In *Advances in Plant Biopesticides* ed. Singh D., editor. (New Delhi: Springer;), 47–62.

Tavares, W. S., Costa, M. A., Cruz, I., Silveira, R. D., Serrão, J. E., and Zanuncio, J. C. (2010). "The Selective effects of natural and synthetic insecticides on mortality of *Spodoptera frugiperda* (Lepidoptera: Noctuidae) and its predator *Eriopis connexa* (Coleoptera: Coccinellidae)." *J. Environ. Sci. Health B.* 45:557–561.

Timmins, W.A., and Reynolds, S.F. (1992). "Azadirachtin inhibits secretion of trypsin in midgut of *Manduca sexta* caterpillars: reduced growth due to impaired protein digestion." *Entomol. Exp Appl.* 63:47-54.

Trumm, P. and Dorn, A. (2000). "Effects of azadirachtin on the regulation of midgut peristalsis by the stomatogastric nervous system in *Locusta migratoria*." *Phytoparasitica* 28:7-26.

Turner, C.J., M.S. Tempesta, R.B. Taylor, M.G. Zagorski, J.C. Termini, Schroeder,D.R.,and Nakanishi, K.(1987)."An NMR spectroscopic study of azadirachtin and its trimethylether." *Tetrahedron* 43:2789-2803.

Varma, J., and Dubey, N.K. (1999). "Prospectives of botanical and microbial products as pesticides of tomorrow." *Curr Sci (India)* 76:172-179.

Venkateswarlu, B., Pirat, M., Kishore, N., and Rasul, A. (2008). "Mycorrhizal inoculation in neem (*Azadirachta indica*) enhances azadirachtin content in seed kernels." *World J. Microbiol. Biotechnol* 24:1243–1247.

Walter, J. F. (1999). "Commercial experience with neem products" In: F.R. Hall and J.J. Menn (eds.), *Biopesticides use and delivery*. Humana, Totowa, N.J 155-170.

Ward, S.M., Delaquis, P.J., Holley, R.A., and Mazza, G. (1998). Inhibition of spoilage and pathogenic bacteria on agar and pre-cooked roasted beef by volatile horse radish distillates. *Food Res Int* 31: 19-26.

Weathersbee, A. A., and McKenzie, C. L. (2005). "Effect of a neem biopesticide on repellency, mortality, oviposition, and development of diaphorina citri (homoptera: psyllidae)." *Fla. Entomol.* 88:401–407.

Wijewardane, R.M.N.A., and Guleria, S.P.S. (2009). *Combined Effects of Pre-cooling, Application of Natural Extracts and Packaging on the*

Storage Quality of Apple (Malus domestica) cv. Royal Delicious 21: 10-20.

Wilps, H., Kirkilionis, E., and Muschenich, K. (1992). "The effects of neem oil and azadirachtin on mortality, flight activity, and energy metabolism of *Schistocerca gregaria* forskal — A comparison between laboratory and field locusts." *Comp. Biochem. Physiol. C Comp. Pharmacol.* 102:67–71.

Xu, J., Fan, Q. J., Yin, Z. Q., Li, X. T., Du, Y. H., and Jia, R.Y., et al. (2010). "The preparation of neem oil microemulsion (*Azadirachta indica*) and the comparison of acaricidal time between neem oil microemulsion and other formulations in vitro." *Vet. Parasitol.* 169:399–403.

Yang, R. Z., and Tang, C.S. (1987). "Plants used for pest control in China." A literature review, *Econ.Bot*42:376-406.

In: Seed Oil
Editor: Nguyen Khanh Dieu Hong
ISBN: 978-1-53613-560-2

Chapter 3

UTILIZATION OF *CALOPHYLLUM INOPHYLLUM* SEED OIL

Setiyo Gunawan[1,*], Hakun Wirawasista Aparamarta[1] and Yi-Hsu Ju[2]

[1]Department of Chemical Engineering Institut Teknologi Sepuluh Nopember, Surabaya, Indonesia
[2]Department of Chemical Engineering National Taiwan University of Science and Technology, Taipei, Taiwan

ABSTRACT

Calophyllum inophyllum is a mangrove plant species from the family of *Calophyllaceae*. It is a native of southern coastal India to Malesia, northern Australia, East Africa, and the Pacific Islands. It produces fruits at age of 7-58 years. Fruit and seed productions are 60-220 and 50-150 kg/tree/year, respectively. Most researchers were focused on conversion of *C. inophyllum* oil into biodiesel due to its high oil content. Therefore, the aim of this chapter is to discuss the production, refining, and

* Corresponding Author Email: gunawan@chem-eng.its.ac.id.

utilization of *C. inophyllum* seed oil as well as its future perspective. Oil content (%) and yield (kg oil per ha) of several edible and non-edible oils were presented. The development of new refining techniques of *C. inophyllum* seed oil has gained increasing importance in the biodiesel and pharmaceutical industries, due to its content of economically-valuable compounds, the necessity of environmental friendly process, and energy security. There are several different methodologies of separation and purification for improving the quality of *C. inophyllum* oil purity (triacylglycerol), such as chemical, physical and batchwise solvent-solvent extraction. Moreover, fatty acids in triacylglycerol (TAG) are the key factor for the quality of oil due to the *cis* and *trans* configuration. It is of great interest if new utilization of *C. inophyllum* seed oil is available. This oil may have a potential to be used as an edible oil after treatments. However, further clinical studies are needed.

Keywords: *C. inophyllum, cis-trans* configuration, fatty acid, refining, triglyceride

Introduction

World energy and food demands are expected to increase due to the expanding urbanization, better living standards, and increasing population. At a time when society is getting increasingly aware of the declining reserves of fossil fuels besides the environmental concerns, it has become apparent that the biofuel is destined to serve a substantial contribution to the future energy of the domestic and industrial economies. Recently, the feedstocks of biodiesel are edible oils, such as sunflower, rapeseed and palm oils. The use of an edible oil to fulfill energy demand induces problems like the sustainability of this practice due to its competition with food, land, and water (Kansedo et al., 2009; Santacesaria et al., 2012). The other reasons might cause food shortage especially in developing countries and environmental problems due to the use available of arable land to produce oil crops (Atabani et al., 2013). Therefore, non-edible oils as the second generation of feedstocks become more attractive for the biodiesel production to fulfill energy demand but will not compete with food. Moreover, the use of non-edible oil for biodiesel production can decrease the biodiesel production cost (Berchmans and Hirata, 2008). This is because the non-edible oils are cheap.

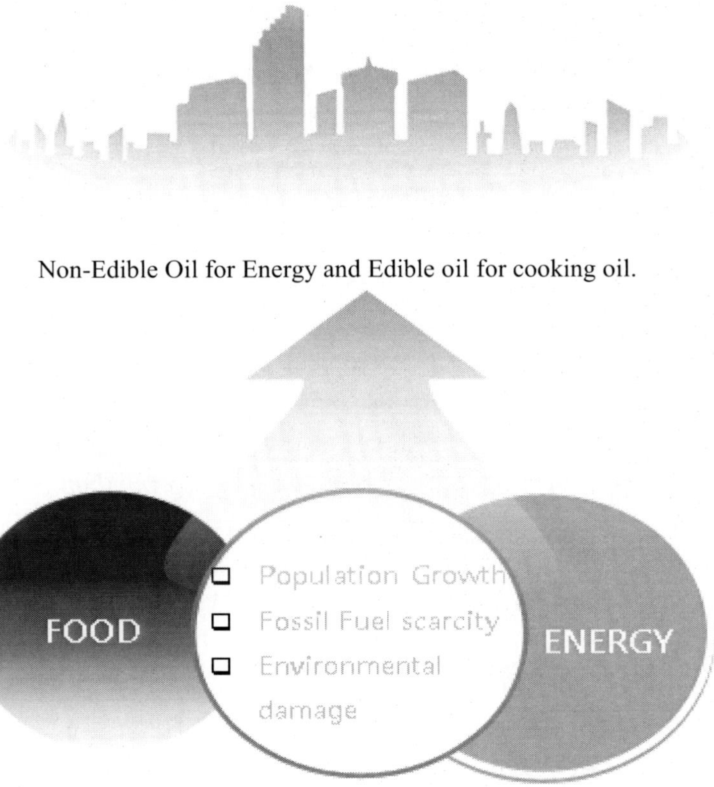

Figure 1. Food and energy competition.

Recent comprehensive reviews on biodiesel production from various feedstocks show the advantages of non-edible oils over edible oils. Production of biodiesel from non-edible oil feedstocks can overcome the problems of food versus fuel, environmental and economic issues related to the edible vegetable oils (Gui, 2008). Moreover, the use of non-edible feedstocks for biodiesel production could provide some leeway such as economic and environmental sustainability, will not compete with food and these crops can thrive on marginal lands (Atabani et al., 2013). Some non-edible oils are even drought-resistant thereby eliminating any potential conflict with water supply. Some examples of non-edible oil seed crops are

Jatropha curcas, Calophyllum inophyllum, Sterculia feotida, Madhuca indica (mahua), *Pongamia glabra* (koroch seed), *linseed, Pongamia pinnata* (Karanja), *Hevea brasiliensis* (rubber seed), *Azadirachta indica* (neem), *Camelina sativa, Lesquerella fendleri, Nicotiana tabacum* (tobacco), *Deccan hemp, Ricinus communis L.* (castor), *Babassu, Simmondsia chinensis* (jojoba), *Eruca sativa. L* and *Xilocarpus moluccensis* (Atabani et al., 2013; Gunawan et al., 2014).

FRUIT, SEED, AND OIL PRODUCTION

The *Calophyllum* genus is a tropical plant that consists of 180-200 different species that are famous for rich in a number of bioactive compounds (Su et al, 2008). One species of the *Calophyllum* genus is *Calophyllum inophyllum Lin* (*C. inophyllum*). *C. inophyllum* is a native of East Africa, southern coastal India to Malesia, northern Australia, and the Pacific islands. The species is widespread along the coasts of eastern Africa (from Kenya to northern Mozambique), Madagascar and other Indian Ocean islands, southeast Asia, northern Australia, north Queensland and the islands of the Pacific Ocean (Lim, 2012).

In Indonesia, it spreads especially in the coastal areas, such as National Parks Alas Purwo, Kepulauan Seribu, Baluran, Ujung Kulon, Nature Reserve Pananjung Pangandaran, Batu Karas Regions, Carita Beach Banten, Yapen, Jayapura, Biak, Nabire, Manokwari, Sorong, Fak Fak (Papua region), Halmahera and Ternate (North Maluku) and Berbak (West Coast of Sumatra) as can be seen in Table 1. *C. inophyllum* plants grow in sandy coastal areas that are marginal and tolerant of salinity and soil with a pH of 4 to 7.4 (Forestry Department, 2008). *C. inophyllum* produces fruits at age 7-58 years (Bustomi et al., 2008). Fruit and seed productions are 60-220 and 50-150 kg/tree/year, respectively. The variability of fruit and seed production was attributed to *C. inophyllum* cultivar, harvesting age, and diversity of agronomic factors.

C. inophyllum has become one of the promising sources of non-edible oils. This is because *C. inophyllum* has high oil content and yield as can be seen in Table 2. Oil yield and oil content of a crop became the key factor to decide the suitability of a crop as the feedstock for biodiesel production. The reason is oil crops with higher oil yield can reduce the production cost. Generally, the cost of raw materials accounts for about 70–80% of the total production cost of biodiesel (Gui et al., 2008).

Table 1 *C. inophyllum* fruit and seed production in several locations in Indonesia

No	Location	Fruit Production (kg/plant/years)	Seed Production (kg/plant/years)
1	Batukaras, Ciamis[1]	60-110	40-80
2	Segara Anakan Block, TN Alas Purwo, Banyuwangi[2]	220	150
3	Ketawang Beach, KPH Purworejo	70-150	50-100
4	Yapen, Papua[1)]	130	90

[1] BPK Ciamis and BPK Manokwari.

[2] Perum Perhutani KPH Purworejo.

Table 2. Source of non-edible vegetable oil

Feedstock	Source	Oil Content (Wt%)	Yields (Kg oil/ ha)	Reference
Annona squamosa	seed	15-20	-	Wirawan, 2008
Balanites aegyptiaca	kernel	36-47	-	Chapagain et al., 2009
C. inophyllum	Seed	40-73	4680	Singh, 2010
Croton tiglium	Seed	30-45	-	Azamm et al., 2005
Cuphea	Seed	20-38	900	Berti & Johnson, 2005
Crotalaria retusa L.	seed	15	-	Umerie et al., 2010
Garcinia indica	seed	45.5	-	No SY, 2011
Guizotia abyssinica L. (niger)	seed	50-60	200-300	Umerie et al., 2010
Jatropha curcas L.	seed	20-60	1590	Sahoo et al., 2007
Madhuca indica	seed	35-50	-	Azamm et al., 2005
Melia azedarach	Seed	10-45	-	Jean, 2011

Table 3. Source of edible vegetable oil

Feedstock	Source	Oil Content (Wt%)	Yields (Kg oil/ ha)	References
Soybean	Seed	18-20	375	Langstraat, 1976; Pryde, 1980; Hoffmann, 1989;
Palm	fruit	42	5000	Atasie and Akinhamnie, 2009
Rapeseed	seed	41- 46	1000	Cakmakli and Unal, 1988
Corn	Fruit	48	145	Demirbas, 2008
Linseed	Seed	40-44	402	Atabani et al., 2014
Peanut	Seed	45-55	890	Atabani et al., 2014

Another, the various parts of *C. inophyllum* can be used as traditional herbal remedies (Lim, 2012), such as the sap for treating wound, the bark for serving as antiseptic and disinfectant, the root for treating wounds and heart stroke, the leaves for treating eye inflammation (Bruneton, 1993; Lemmens, 2003), and the seed oil for treating rheumatism, producing soap, and healing wound in skin (Dweck and Meadows, 2002). In Indonesia, the half-ripe fruit is pickled but only the seed is eaten. This caution is needed as toxic compounds may be present in the fruit and seed (Burkill et al., 1996).

Table 3 shows the source of edible vegetable oils. As can be seen, palm oil gives the highest oil yield with 5000 kg oil per hectare, considerably higher than other oils which are only in the range of hundreds to 1000 kg oil per hectare. Therefore, the palm oil has become a promising feedstock to fulfill energy demand.

Table 2 and 3 show that *C. inophyllum* (non-edible oil) and palm (edible oil) are potential biofuel feedstock based on their oil content and yield. *C. inophyllum* has one big advantage over palm in that it is non-edible and will not diminish food supply in the developing countries (Atabani et al., 2013).

TOTAL LIPID

The total lipids of *C. inophyllum* consist of 92.0% neutral lipids, 6.4% glycolipids and 1.6% phospholipids. Neutral lipids consist of triacylglycerols (TAG), free fatty acids (FFA) and small amounts of diacylglycerols (DAG), monoacylglycerols (MAG) and sterols. At least four glycolipids and five phospholipids have been identified (Hemavathy and Prabhakar, 1990).

Neutral Lipids

Neutral lipids are conjugates of amphipathic alcohols and fatty acids. Usually, the predominant neutral lipids are TAG as can be seen in Table 4. Free sterols (such as cholesterol, ergosterol, and sitosterol) can be acylated to form steryl esters (SE), whereas TAG is synthesized through the esterification of diacylglycerols. Neutral lipids can be surrounded by a hydrophilic shell composed of phospholipids or serum lipoproteins, they can be encompassed by detergents and phospholipids (intestinal micelles). Neutral lipids can be synthesized by simple commonality reaction (Ruggles et al., 2013). Free alcohols (predominantly sterols and diacylglycerols but also retinols and long-chain alcohols) are conjugated by esterification with fatty acids derived from either acyl-coenzyme A or phospholipids (commonly phosphatidylcholine)

C. inophyllum oil usually contains a large amount of FFA (~5-10 wt.%) as it can be seen in Table 4. Because of this reason, it cannot be converted directly into biodiesel following the conventional alkali-catalyzed transesterification reaction. A two- or three- stage method has been applied to produce high-quality biodiesel from this feedstock by a few researchers. For example, Sahoo et al., (2007) utilized a three-stage transesterification process to produce biodiesel from *C. inophyllum* oil with an initial acid value of 44 mg KOH/g. Also, biodiesel was produced from the oil of *C. inophyllum* via acid pre-treatment, transesterification, and post-treatment stages. FFA level in the oil should be below 3% for alkaline-catalyzed transesterification (Sharma and Singh, 2009; Ribeiro et al., 2011) and below 0.3% for edible oils (SNI 01-3741, 2002).

Quantitative data of lipid fractions of crude oils are shown in Table 4. TAGs are the predominant lipid class in all samples, representing more than 50% for crude oils of *C. inophyllum*; followed by diglyceride (DAG), then FFA.

Venkanna (2009) investigated the properties of *C. inophyllum* oil. This oil has a density of 910 kg/m^3, a kinematic viscosity at 400°C of 32.48 m^2/s, a flash point of 224 ° C, a saponification value of 191-202, an iodine value of 82.98, and an acid value of 4.76 mg KOH/g. The original color of *C. inophyllum* oil is dark green. After saponification, the color becomes bright yellow.

According to Crane et al., (2005), *C. inophyllum* oil contains 70.8% unsaturated fatty acids (70.8%) much higher than saturated fatty acids (29.2%). Aparamarta et al., (2016) reported that crude *C. inophyllum* oil was dominated by 78.30% TAG, 5.35% DAG, and 8.51% free fatty acid. The TAG is the largest content of oil in the *C. inophyllum* which is an ester with glycerol and three fatty acids. The use of non-edible oils as human food is hindered by the presence of toxic components (Ahmad et al., 2011). Moreover, Lee and Gibot (1986) reported that *C. inophyllum* oil can be turned into an edible oil after refinement and detoxification.

Table 4. Composition of crude *C. inophyllum* oil

	Content (Wt%)				
Component	Aparamarta et al., 2016	Rudi Wijaya et al., 2009	Crane et al., 2005	Dweck, 2002	Hemavaty and Prabhakar, 1990
Triacylglycerols	78.30 ± 3.9	54.17	76.70	72.46	74.0
Diacylglycerols	5.35 ± 1.27	4.08	7.00	7.43	6.36
Monoacylglycerols	2.75 ± 0.33	2.97	< 0.1	2.55	3.00
Free fatty acids	8.51 ± 0.31	4.33	5.10	9.16	8.85
Others	2.47 ± 1.25	34.45	11.20	8.41	7.79

Phospholipids

Phospholipids or *phosphatides* are lipids that contain phosphoric acid group in their structure. Phospholipids are diesters of phosphoric acid, H_3PO_4 (Heller et al., 1993). Most phospholipids contain a *diglyceride*, a *phosphate* group, and a simple organic molecule, such as choline as can be seen in Table 5. There are two main kinds of phospholipids: *glycerophospholipids* and *sphingomyelins*. *Glycerophospholipids* are closely related to fats and oils in that they contain a glycerol backbone linked by ester bonds to two fatty acids and one phosphoric acid.

In phospholipids, the phosphate group is hydrophilic, while the two fatty acids are hydrophobic. When phospholipids are mixed with water, they spontaneously reorder themselves to form the lowest free-energy configuration. This means that the hydrophilic regions interact with water, while the hydrophobic regions find ways to move away from water.

Table 5. Phospholipids of *C. inophyllum* kernel[1]

Phospholipids	Content (Wt%)	Fatty acid profile (Wt%)			
		16:00	18:0	18:1	18:2
Lysophosphatidylcholine	5.7	60.4	9.6	7.9	22.1
Phosphatidylserine	6.1	25.5	7.7	23.7	43.1
Phosphatidic acid	8.1	10.0	6.0	33.9	50.1
Phosphatidylcholine	33.8	50.3	9.4	13.5	36.8
Phosphatidylethanolamine	46.3	6.9	7.3	37.6	48.2

[1]Hemavaty and Prabhakar, 1990.

Glycolipids

Glycolipids are a heterogeneous group structure of membrane-bound compounds found in all living organisms from prokaryotic to eukaryotic cells, from bacteria to humans. The term ‘glycolipid’ comprises any compound containing one or more monosaccharides glycosidically linked to a lipid moiety. However, according to newer nomenclature

(IUPAC/IUBMB, 1996), the term 'glycolipid' is to be restricted to acylglycerols, ceramides, and phenols. Glycolipids are essential constituents of cellular membranes and have an enormous number of functions. They are important for cell aggregation or dissociation, they may act as receptors and provide specific contact, and they may deliver or receive signals. Many glycolipids may modulate the immune response, for example, gangliosides and bacterial lipopolysaccharides.

Glycolipids with a glycerol backbone, similar to phosphoglycerides, belong to glycoglycerolipids, usually as diacyl sugars, and those with a sphingosine base belong to the class of cerebrosides and gangliosides as can be seen in Table 6. It is of some interest that several glycolipids, consisting only of fatty acids in combination with carbohydrates, show marked biological activity. No information is available on the mechanism of toxicity of these materials for microorganisms and higher animals.

Table 6. Glycolipids of *C. inophyllum* kernel[1]

Glycolipids	Content (Wt%)	Fatty acid profile (Wt%)			
		16:00	18:0	18:1	18:2
Monogalactosyldiacylglycerol	11.4	28.0	7.9	21.0	43.1
Acylated sterolglucoside	13.1	5.6	7.6	1.3	85.5
Monogalactosylmonoacylglcerol	22.2	20.0	8.2	26.4	45.4
Acylmonogalactosyldiacylglycerol	53.3	12.9	0.1	0.9	86.1

[1]Hemavaty and Prabhakar, 1990.

Fatty Acids of Calophyllum Inophyllum Oil

Fatty acids are long chain molecules of lipid-carboxylic acid discovered in oils and fats, and in cell membranes as a component of phospholipids and glycolipids. The other definition of fatty acids is carbon chains with a methyl group at one end of the molecule (designated omega, ω) and a carboxyl group at the other end (Figure 2). The carbon atom next to the carboxyl group is called the carbon, and the subsequent one the β carbon. The letter n is also often used instead of the Greek ω to indicate the position of the double bond closest to the methyl end. Mjos and Pettersen (2001) reported that the n-6 position is often referred to omega 6 (ω-6) position. This nomenclature was used to di- or poly-unsaturated fatty acid isomers. The systematic nomenclature for fatty acids may also indicate the location of double bonds with reference to the carboxyl group (Δ).

Fatty acids may be named pursuant to systematic or trivial nomenclature. One systematic way to describe fatty acids is related to the methyl (ω) end. This is to describe the position of double bonds from the end of the fatty acid. The letter n is also often used to describe the ω position of double bonds.

Fatty acids of some non-edible oils are generally aliphatic compounds with a carboxyl group at the end of a straight chain. The most common fatty acids are C_{16} and C_{18} acids. However, some feedstocks contain significant amounts of fatty acids other than the typical C_{16} and C_{18} acids (Knothe et al., 2010). Fatty acids represent 30–35% of total energy intake in many industrial countries and the most important dietary sources of fatty acids are vegetable oils, dairy products, meat products, grain and fatty fish or fish oils.

Fatty acids can be classified into saturated fatty acid and unsaturated fatty acid because of the number of hydrogen atoms bonded to carbon atoms as can be seen in Figure 3 (Atabani et al., 2013). Saturated fatty acids are fatty acids in which two hydrogen atoms bonded to a single carbon atom. It said to be saturated because the carbon atoms have the maximum hydrogen binding. This type of fatty acids have no double bonds between the individual carbon atoms of the fatty acid chain. That is, the chain of carbon atoms is fully "saturated" with hydrogen atoms. There are many kinds of naturally occurring saturated fatty acids, which differ mainly in the number of carbon atoms, from 3 (propionic acid) to 36 (hexatriacontanoic acid).

$$\underset{\omega}{CH_3} - (CH_2)_n - CH2 - \underset{\beta}{CH\ 2} - \underset{\alpha}{COOH}$$

Figure 2. Nomenclature for fatty acids.

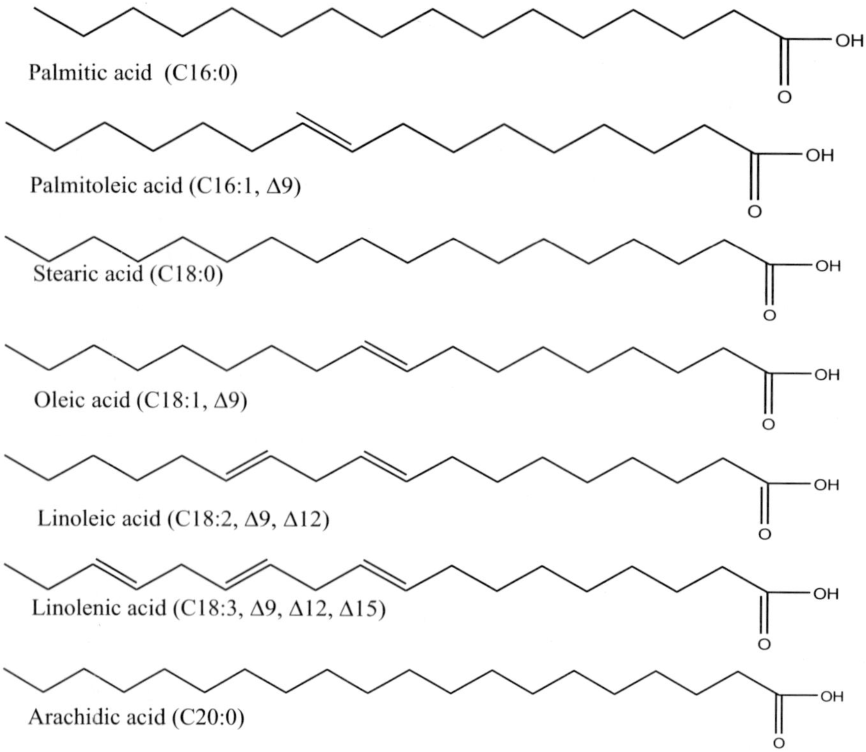

Figure 3. Structure of fatty acids.

Table 7. Fatty acid composition of *C. inophyllum* oil

Fatty Acid		Content (Wt%)				
		Atabani et al. (2013)	Ramaraju and Ashok (2011)	Ajayi et al. (2008)	Sahoo et al. (2006)	Crane et al. (2005)
Palmitic Acid	C16:0	12.01	14.8-18.5	14,6	12.01	13.7
Stearic Acid	C18:0	12.95	6.1-9.2	16,5	12.95	14.3
Oleic Acid	C18:1	34.09	36.2-53.1	39,8	34.09	39.1
Linoleic Acid	C18:2	38.26	15.8-28.5	27,6	38.26	31.1
Linolenic Acid	C18:3	0.30	NA	0,38	0.30	0.3
Arachidic Acid	C20:0	NA[a]	NA	NA	NA	0.6
Behenic Acid	C22:0	NA	NA	NA	NA	0.2

[a]Not Available.

The other is unsaturated fatty acids. It is called unsaturated fatty acid because it has the double bond. In this case, the carbon atoms of the hydrogen atom are fully bound with hydrogen because of the double bond. Saturated fatty acids and unsaturated fatty acids are different in that they have different energy and melting point. Because unsaturated fatty acids contain fewer carbon-hydrogen bond than saturated fatty acids with the same number of carbon atoms, unsaturated fatty acids have less energy during metabolism than saturated fatty acids.

Polyunsaturated fatty acids in plant oils have the ability to heal wounds (Lamer, 1962; Bowman, 1980; Gibson, 1983; Grubauer et al., 1989). The healing power of *C. inophyllum* oil is partly derived from its polyunsaturated fatty acids. Table 7 shows the fatty acid composition of *C. inophyllum* oil reported by several researchers. It can be seen that crude *C. inophyllum* oil is dominated by C18:1 followed by C18:2, C18:0, and C16:0. The percentage and type of fatty acids composition of *C. inophyllum* oil vary depending on the quality of feedstock, growth conditions and geographical location in which the plant was grown (Atabani and Cesar, 2014).

Trans **and** ***Cis*** **Fatty Acid in Triglyceride of** ***Calophyllum inophyllum*** **Oil**

The TAG is the major component in *C. inophyllum* oil which is an ester with glycerol and three fatty acids. Some fatty acids have benefit for human health. One of them is *cis* oleic acid. This fatty acid has benefits, such as protection from free radicals and other oxidative stressors (Haug et al., 2007), reducing blood pressure while increasing good HDL cholesterol in women (Ruiz-Gutiérrez et al., 1996), and cancer preventive (Elezabeth and Arumugam, 2014). The TAG may also be harmful to human health and may cause problems, such as cardiovascular disease, cancer, obesity, and diabetes (Berquin et al., 2008). One of the reason is the content of *trans* fatty acids in the oil. Therefore, *cis* and *trans* fatty acids configuration in TAG play a critical role in the determining quality of an edible oil.

Trans fatty acid (TFA) is an unsaturated fatty acid with at least one double bond in the trans configuration. It's produced artificially by heating liquid vegetable oils into shortening and margarine. The most common TFA is monounsaturated, but various di-unsaturated *cis*, *trans* and *trans*, *cis* isomers also occur. In *trans* monounsaturated fatty acids of partially hydrogenated oil, the double bond tends to be normally distributed around positions 9 to 11 with a range of 5 to 15 (Dutton, 1979; Marchand, 1982). Because of the presence of double bonds in aliphatic hydrocarbon chain of unsaturated fatty acids, they can exhibit geometrical isomerism also called as *cis-trans* isomerization. Naturally, occurring fatty acid exhibits *cis*-configuration which can be modified to *trans* configuration. In *cis*-form the hydrogen atoms of double bonded carbon atom oriented on the same side, however in *the trans* form they oriented in opposite direction as can be seen in Figure 4. The difference in geometry of *trans* and *cis*-unsaturated fatty acid plays an important role in the biological function of the fatty acid.

Cis and *trans* forms of fatty acids show different physical and chemical properties just like other organic geometrical isomers as can be seen in Table 8. *Trans* isomers show a higher melting point due to closely packed structure than *cis* isomers (De Greyt et al., 1999). Consumption of TFAs is considered unsafe because it can be responsible for the cardiovascular disease (Judd et al., 1994).

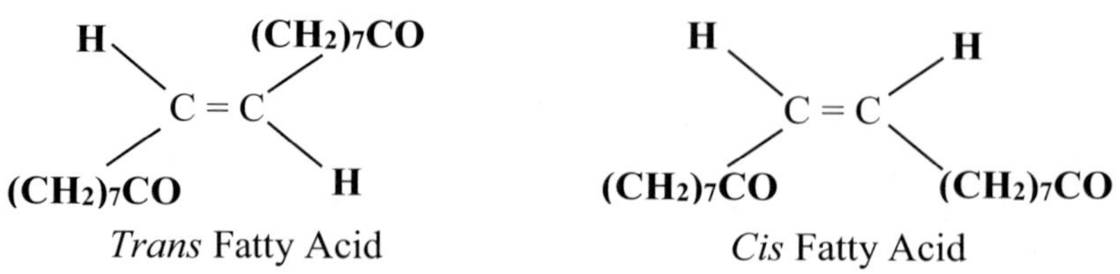

Figure 4. Trans and *cis* fatty acids.

Table 8. Difference between *cis* and *trans* fatty acids[1]

Properties	*Cis* Fatty Acid	*Trans* Fatty Acid
Health Effect	Good	Detrimental, increases the level of bad cholesterol in the body
Natural Occurrence	Yes	Very rare, hence produced artificially by partial hydrogenation of polyunsaturated fatty acid
Orientation at double bonded carbon atoms	Hydrogen atoms at double bonded carbon atoms on the same side	Hydrogen atoms at double bonded carbon atoms on the opposite side
Recommended consumption	Can be consumed as per requirement	No more than 1% of total calories per day
Commonly found in	Natural fatty acids	Processed food, fast foods, butter and milk products
Melting point	Lower	Higher

[1]Hemavaty and Prabhakar, 1990; FAO, 2008.

In western, the level of TFA is about 6% of the fat or 7 gram/day in a total fat intake of 120 gram/day for diet (FAO, 1994). A group in Harvard Medical School reported that TFA was allowed in the human body only 2 to 7 gram/day or below than 6% of the total fat intake (FAO, 1994). Another issue is the resemblance of *trans*-fatty acid to saturated fatty acids in the structure which can interrupt many biochemical reactions.

In general, three different dietary sources of TFA can be distinguished: ruminant fats, partially hydrogenated fats, and refined oils. Ruminant fats are the only natural source of TFA with vaccenic acid (11-*trans* 18:1) as the predominant one. On the other hand, partially hydrogenated fats are known as the major dietary source of TFA. Besides saturation of double bonds, partial hydrogenation is also characterized by the positional and geometrical isomerization of double bonds, resulting in a large amount of *trans* 18:1 isomers. Refined oils contain only a limited amount of TFA, mainly *trans* 18:2 and 18:3 isomers formed during deodorization. Other differences between *cis* and *trans*-fatty acids can be seen in Table 8.

REFINING PROCESS

The biggest challenge in using crude *C. inophyllum* oil as the biodiesel feedstock is that it is prone to saponification reaction leading to soap formation during alkaline-catalyzed transesterification. The saponification reaction makes the reduction of biodiesel yields because of the reducing of the biodiesel formation rate (Saraf and Thomas, 2007; Thiruvengadaravi et al., 2012). This is because crude *C. inophyllum* oil usually contains a large amount of free fatty acids. FFA level in the oil should be below the desired level, less than 3% for alkaline-catalyzed transesterification, (Sharma and Singh, 2009; Ribeiro et al., 2011) and less than 0.3% for edible oils (SNI 01-3741, 2002). Therefore, degumming, neutralization, bleaching, and deodorization steps are applied in the isolating of triacylglycerols that are used as a feedstock of biodiesel production (refined vegetable oil).

Chemical Refining

Chemical/alkali refining consists of the following steps: degumming, neutralization, bleaching, and deodorization as can be seen in Figure 5. The summarization of the chemical, physical refining, and batchwise solvent-solvent extraction can be seen in Table 9.

The first step of a chemical refining is degumming. Its purpose is to remove seed particles, impurities, gum and most of the phosphatides, carbohydrates, proteins, and traces of metals (Carr, 1976). For acid degumming, it reduces calcium and magnesium by 88 and 90%, respectively (Zufarov et al., 2008). Iron and fatty acid are also reduced. Iron can be reduced from 4.4 to 3.3 ppm (Karaali, 1985) and from 1.24 to 0.23 wt.% (Kreps et al., 2014). This step is also effective in the reducing desirable molecules, such as tocopherols. Moreover, the total content of linoleic acid and high oleic sunflower oil can be reduced to 6.6% and 8.4%, respectively (Kreps et al., 2014).

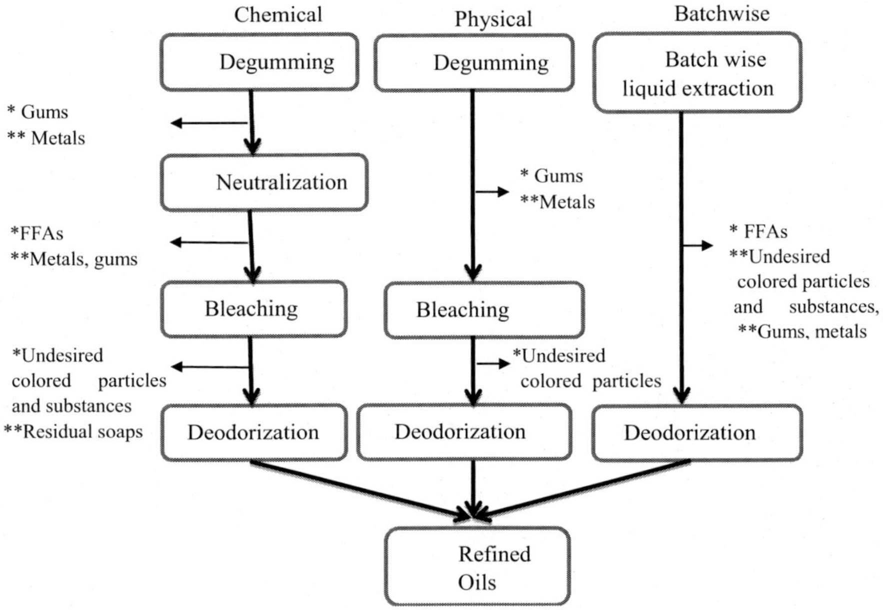

Figure 5. Refining steps of vegetable oils.

The neutralization step decreases the content of FFAs and their oxidation products, part of the pigments, traces of metals, residual proteins, phosphatides, and carbohydrates. Mallah et al., (2011) reported that oil content can be increased from 96.0 to 96.4% in the chemically refined cottonseed oil. The increased oil content is due to the decreasing of other components, such as FFA and DAG which were decreased from 1.0 to 0.1 and 2.9 to 2.5, respectively.

The purpose of bleaching (or decolorizing) is to reduce the levels of pigments, such as carotenoids and chlorophyll, but it also further removes residues of phosphatides, soaps, traces of metals, oxidation products, and proteins. These must be reduced in order to improve the quality of the final product. This step did not decrease the FFA content in sunflower oil (Kreps et al., 2014). Mallah et al., (2011) reported that the oil content was increased from 96.4 to 96.7% in this step. The other component, such as DAG and FFA were decreased from 2.5 to 2.4% and 0.1 to 0.03%, respectively.

Table 9. Summary of comparison between chemical and physical refinings and batchwise solvent-solvent extraction

Feed	Method	Result	Reference
Cottonseed Oil	Chemical refining	TAG content increased from 96.0 to 99.36 DAG, MAG, FFA content decreased from 2.9 to 0.5, 0.1 to 0.08 and 1 to 0.06, respectively	Mallah et al., 2011
C. inophyllum seed oil	Batchwise solvent-solvent extraction	TAG content increased from 78.53 to 98.53 DAG, and FFA content decreased from 5.35 to 0.42, 8.51 to 0.53, respectively	Aparamarta et al. , 2016
Sunflower oil	Chemical refining	14-34% loss of total tocopherols	Alpaslan et al., 2001; Talal et al., 2013; Ergönül and Köseoˇglu, 2014.
Sunflower oil	Chemical refining	60.3% loss of total phytosterols	Karaali, 1985; Nergiz and Çelikkale, 2011
Sunflower oil	Physical refining	ND loss of total phytosterols	Tasan and Demirci, 2005; Kreps et al., 2014
Sunflower oil	Physical refining	24.6-54.8% loss of total tocopherols	Tasan and Demirci, 2005; Kreps et al., 2014

The final step is deodorization. In this step, the relatively volatile components of FFA that give rise to undesirable flavors, colors and odors in fats and oils are removed (Akterian, 2009). This step improves the taste, odor, flavor, color and the stability of the oil. Gotor and Razi (2016) used this method to remove contaminants (pesticides and process solvents) and other compounds (tocopherols) that could hamper the continuity of the chemical refining process and the quality of the product. Total tocopherol content gradually declined from 5.85 to 3.6%. The oil content was significantly increased from 96.7 to 99.36% (Mallah et al., 2011).

Physical Refining

Physical refining differs from the chemical refining only in that it does not have a neutralization step. After degumming, it directly goes to bleaching. Alpaslan et al., (2001) used this method to reduce total tocopherols in the sunflower crude oil. This method resulted in a higher reduction of total tocopherol content than the chemical refining process. Total tocopherols loss during physical refining varied from 24.6 to 54.8% with an average loss of 41% (Alpaslan et al., 2001; Tasan and Demirci, 2005; Kreps et al., 2014).

Batchwise Solvent-Solvent Extraction

Extraction is a relatively new method in the chemical engineering. This method is used to separate the desired substance when mixed with other substances. The mixture is brought into contact with a solvent in which the desired substance will dissolve, but the other substances present in the solution will be insoluble. Gunawan et al., (2008) reported that binary solvent extraction provides better separation of fatty acid steryl esters with higher purity and recovery when applied to lipid fraction with a high initial fatty acid steryl esters content. This method has some advantages like environmental friendly because of the solvents can be recovered easily and less sophisticated equipment.

Aparamarta et al., (2016) explained that the crude oil was separated into two fractions based on differences in polarity of the constituent components by single-stage and multi-stage solvent extraction (batch-wise solvent extraction). It was based on the principle of distribution of a substance between a polar solvent (methanol) and a non-polar solvent (hexane or petroleum ether). The effects of various factors on the separation, such as of solvent to oil mass ratio, solvent mixture and methanol content in the solvent mixture were systematically investigated.

Crude C. inophyllum oil was dark green and viscous at room temperature. After multistage stirred batch-wise solvent-solvent extraction, it was separated into bright yellow non-polar lipids fraction (NPLF) and dark green polar lipid fraction (PLF). The color change of NPLF may be caused by its increased TAG content. The content of TAG in NPLF was increased from 78.3 to 98.53 wt%. However, the PLF color remained the same as crude oil. Moreover, xanthone was detected in the crude oil which can be used for medical purposes such as the anti-HIV virus (Aparamarta et al., 2016). Xanthone probably is toxic compound that makes the PLF color was not change

UTILIZATION OF *C. INOPHYLLUM*

C. inophyllum is a mangrove plant species from the family of *Calophyllaceae*. Among mangrove seed oils, *C. inophyllum* oil is becoming an important raw material for biodiesel production. This is because *C. inophyllum* has a high oil content (40-73%) and yield (4680 kg oil per ha) (Atabani et al., 2013). Therefore, an alternative way to achieve development of mangrove areas is an utilization of *C. inophyllum* as low-cost material for producing biodiesel and pharmaceutical products.

Biodiesel

Recently, the use of vegetable oils falls into two applications namely: a) food industry, and b) industrial uses, including biodiesel. FAO (2013) reported that the use of edible oil is for food and biodiesel. Thus, the rapidly growing demand for vegetable oils has been triggered by the food market rather than the industrial or biodiesel market. In the food industry, vegetable oil is used for human food, such as margarine, baking and frying fats or shortening (Alston et al., 2002). Therefore, non-edible oils as the second generation of feedstocks become more attractive for biodiesel production to fulfill energy demand but will not compete with food.

Biodiesel has recognized increasing attention worldwide as a blending component or a direct replacement for diesel fuel in vehicle engines.

Biodiesel, as an alternative fuel for internal combustion engines, is defined as a mixture of monoalkyl esters of long chain fatty acids (FAME) derived from a renewable lipid feedstock, such as vegetable oil or animal fat. Recently, about 84% the world biodiesel production is met by rapeseed oil. The remaining portion is from sunflower oil (13%), palm oil (1%) and soybean oil and others (2%) (Thoenes, 2007). Biodiesel typically contains alkyl fatty acid (chain length C14–C22) esters of short-chain alcohols, primarily, methanol or ethanol. It is the best candidate for diesel fuels in diesel engines. The higher heating values (HHVs) of biodiesels are relatively high. The HHVs of biodiesels (39–41 MJ/kg) are slightly lower than those of gasoline (46 MJ/kg), petrodiesel (43 MJ/kg), or petroleum (42 MJ/kg), but higher than coal (32–37 MJ/kg) (Demirbas, 2008).

The quality of biodiesel fuel can be influenced by various factors, such as the quality of feedstock, the fatty acid composition of the feedstock, type of production and refining process employed and post-production parameters. Therefore, it is required a standard and characteristic of biodiesel fuel. The establishment of standardization for biodiesel has to be wholly owned by many countries. It is utilized to protect both biodiesel consumers and producers as well as to support the development of biodiesel industries. All alternative biodiesel fuels should meet the international standard specification of biodiesel. The biodiesel standards are ASTM6571 and EN14214. These standards describe the physical and chemical characteristics of variety biodiesel produced from non-edible and edible oil resources. Some of these properties include caloric value (MJ/kg), cetane number, density (kg/m^3), viscosity(mm^2/s), cloud and pour points (°C), flashpoint (°C), acid value (mg KOH per g-oil), ash content (%), copper corrosion, carbon residue, water content and sediment, distillation range, sulfur content, glycerin (%m/m), phosphorus (mg/kg), and oxidation stability [Uriarte, 2010; Atadashi et al., 2010; Masjuki, 2010; Sandford, 2011).

For the production of first generation biodiesel, edible vegetable oils, such as soybean, rapeseed, and palm oils are used as the main feedstock. However, the use of edible oils as the energy source has raised a lot of objections from the public and non-government organizations. Thus, the second generation biodiesel produced from non-edible oils, such as *Jatropha curcas L.* appeared as an attractive alternative feedstock for the biodiesel industry. In fact, the use of jatropha oil in existing biodiesel plant does not require major modification of the equipment and process flow, mainly because the oil has similar properties to edible oils. Another advantage of using jatropha oil is that jatropha trees can grow easily on non-arable or wasteland. However, jatropha oil does contain a higher concentration of free fatty acid (FFA) that may require an additional pre-treatment.

Pharmaceutical Products

C. inophyllum oil has been used traditionally as a local medicine, in some island, such as African, Pacific, and Asian. All parts of the plant (bark, leaves, and seeds) have been used medicinally as antiseptics, astringents, expectorants, diuretics, and purgatives. The oils of the seed and root have been used to cure wounds and scabies. In Pacific island folk medicine, the oil has been topically applied to treat various ailments, such as cuts, scrapes, blisters, burns, insect bites and stings, abrasions, acne and acne scars, anal fissures, diabetic sores, dry or scaly skin, eczema, herpes sores, sunburn, psoriasis, and to reduce foot and body odor. The oil has also been topically applied to the neck area to treat a sore throat. The oil is valued for its analgesic and pain-relieving properties and has been used to treat neuralgia, rheumatism, and sciatica. The oil is used in Chinese traditional medicine to treat rheumatism, skin infections, wounds, leprous nephritis, pain, eye diseases, and inflammation. (Ali et al., 1999; Dweck and Meadows, 2002; Shen et al., 2003; Kilham, 2004).

Anti-Bacterial Activity

When *C. inophyllum* oil is applied to wounds in the skin, it has the ability to promote the formation of new tissue. Pacific Islanders use tamanu for treating all sorts of scrapes, burns, rashes, insect bites, psoriasis, scars, and sunburns. Yimdjo et al. (2004) reported that dose of 20 mcg/disc in an agar well diffusion assay, caloxanthone A, calophynic acid, brasiliensic acid, inophylloidic acid, calophyllolide, and inophyllum C and E, were found to hamper *Staphylococcus aureus* but not *Vibrio anguillarium*, *Escherichia coli*, and the yeast *Candida tropicalis*. All of the xanthone compounds in tamanu have anti-inflammatory activity and have been shown to reduce swelling and irritation with topical application.

Anti-Inflammatory Activity

All of the xanthone compounds in *C. inophyllum* have anti-inflammatory activity (Fylaktakidou et al., 2004) and have been proven to reduce swelling and irritation with topical application. *Calophyllolide* isolated from the seed oil has been found in studies to reduce histamine related the inflammation and swelling of tissues along with illophyllide, another active component. Tsai et al., (2012) were studied to evaluate the anti-inflammatory effects of *C. inophyllum* in macrophage cells under lipopolysaccharide (LPS) exposure. Given that this oil has the strong anti-inflammatory properties.

Anti-Oxidant Activity

Pacific Islanders regularly use *C. inophyllum* oil to comfort sunburns due to its regenerative effects. The xanthones and coumarins in the oil are also potent antioxidants and hamper the breakdown of cell membranes from free radicals. One of the most common sources of free radicals in our daily lives is exposure to UV rays from the sun. *C. inophyllum* can help to counteract aging caused by UV related free radicals. Prasad et al., (2012) reported that *C inophyllum* extract leaf showed a good antioxidants activity.

In one study from the European Journal of Pharmaceutical Sciences in 2007, *C. inophyllum* oil was investigated as a UV filter. It was proven to exhibit significant UV absorption capabilities and had a sun protection factor of 18 to 22 even at low concentrations. About 85% of the DNA damage caused by UV exposure was inhibited with just a 1% tamanu oil preparation and was deemed gentle enough to even be used in the eyes as a UV filter.

References

Ahmad, A. L., Mat Yasin, N. H., Derek, C. J. C., Lim, J. K. 2011. Microalgae as a sustainable energy source for biodiesel production: a review. *Renew. Sustain. Energy Rev.* 15, 584–93.

Ali, M. S., Mahmud, S., Perveen, S., Ahmad, V. U., Rizwani, G. H., 1999. Epimers from the leaves of *Calophyllum inophyllum*. *Phytochemistry.* 50,1385-1389.

Alpaslan, M., Tepe, S., Simsek, O. 2001. Effect of refining processes on the total and individual tocopherol content in sunflower oil. *Int. J. Food Sci. Technol*. 36, 737-739.

Alston, J. M., Chalfant, J. A., Piggott, N. E. 2002. Estimating and testing the compensated double-log demand model. *Appl. Econ*. 34, 1177-186.

Atabani, A. E., Cesar, A. D. 2014. *Calophyllum Inophyllum* L. – A prospective non-edible biodiesel feedstock. Study of biodiesel production, properties, fatty acid composition, blending and engine performance. *Renew. Sust. Energ. Rev.* 37, 644-655.

Atabani, A. E., Silitonga, A. S., Ong, H. C., Mahlia, T. M. I., Masjuki, H. H., Badruddin, I. A., Fayaz, H., 2013. Non-edible vegetable oils: A critical evaluation of oil extraction, fatty acid compositions, biodiesel production, characteristics, engine performance and emissions production. *Renew. Sust. Energ. Rev.*, 18, 211–245.

Atasie, V. N., Akinhanmi, T. F., 2009. Extraction, compositional studies and physicochemical characteristics of palm kernel oil. *Pak. J. Nutr.*, 8, 800-803.

Atadashi, I. M., Aroua, M. K., Abdul, A. A. 2010. High-quality biodiesel and its diesel engine application: a review. *Renew. Sust. Energ. Rev.*, 14, 1999–2008.

Ajayi, I. A., Oderinde, R. A., Taiwo, V. O., Agbidana, E. O. 2008. Short-term toxicological evaluation of *Terminalia catappa, Pentaclethra macrophylla* and *Calophyllum inophyllum* seed oil in rats. *Food Chem.*, 106, 458-465.

Azam, M. M., Waris, A., Nahar, N. M. 2005. Prospects and potential of fatty acid methyl esters of some non-traditional seed oils for use as biodiesel in India. *Biomass Bioenerg.*, 29, 293–302.

Aparamarta, W. H., Saputra, T., Claratika, A., Ju, Y. H., Gunawan, S. 2016. Separation and Purification of Triacylglycerols from Nyamplung (*Calophyllum inophyllum*) Oil by Batchwise Solvent Extraction. *Ind Eng Chem Res*, 55, 3113–3119.

Aparamarta, W. H., Ismawan, R., Anggraeni, V., Widjaja, T., Qadariyah, L., Ju, Y. H., Gunawan, S. 2016. Separation and Purification of Xanthones from Polar Fraction Nyamplung (*Calophyllum Inophyllum*) Leaf. *International Symposium for Young Chemical Engineers*, Taiwan.

Baker, J. L. 2008. *Impacts of financial, food, and fuel crisis on the urban poor*, Directions in Urban Development, December, The World Bank, Washington, DC.

Barve, J. A., Okuyama, H., William E. M., Lands, Frank, D. 1972. Gunstone, Selective transfers of trans-ethylenic acids by acyl coenzyme A. Phospholipid acyltransferases. *Biochemistry,* 11, 4392–4398.

Berchmans, H. J., Hirata, S. 2008. Biodiesel production from crude *Jatropha curcas* L. seed oil with a high content of free fatty acids. *Bioresour. Technol.*, 99, 1716–21.

Bowman, W. C. 1980. *Text Book of Pharmacology*. (2nd Edn.). Oxford, U. K: Black well Scientific Publication.

Berquin, I. M., Edwards, I. J., Chen, Y. Q. 2008. Multi-targeted therapy of cancer by omega-3 fatty acids. *Cancer Lett.*, 269, 363–377.

Berti, M. T., Johnson, B. L. 2008. Physiological changes during seed development of cuphea. *Field Crops Res*. 106, 163-170.

Brauner, A., Budzikiewicz, H., Boland, W. 1982. Studies in chemical ionization mass spectrometry. 5. Localization of homoconjugated triene and tetraene units in aliphatic compounds. *Org. Mass Spectrom*., 17, 161-164.

Bruneton, J. 1993. *Plantes Medicinales, Technique and Documents Lavoisier*, 2nd edition; Pharmacognosie–Phytochime: Paris, p 300.

Burkill, I. H., Birtwistle. W., Foxworthy, F. W., Scrivenor, J. B., Watson, J. G. 1966. *A dictionary of the economic products of the Malay Peninsula*; Ministry of Agriculture and Cooperatives: Kuala Lumpur, 1241.

Bustomi, S., Tati Rostiwati, T., Sudradjat, R., Leksono, B., Kosasih, S., Anggraeni, I., Syamsuwida, D., Lisnawati, Y., Mile, Y., Djaenudin, D., Mahfudz, Rachman, E. 2008. *Nyamplung (Calophyllum inophyllum L.). Sumber Energi Biofuel yang Potensial*. [Potential Biofuel Energy Source] Jakarta: Badan Litbang Kehutanan.

Çakmakli, Ü., Ünal, M. K. 1988. Composition and mineral distribution of rapeseed varieties tested for adaptation in turkey. *Fat. Sci. Technol.,* 10, 386-389.

Carr, R. A. 1976. Degumming and refining practices in the U. S. *J. Am. Oil Chemists Soc*. 53, 347-352.

Chapagain, B. P., Yehoshua, Y., Wiesman, Z. 2009. Desert date (*Balanites aegyptiaca*) as an arid land sustainable bioresource for biodiesel. *Bioresour. Technol*. 100, 1221–6.

Crane, S., Aurore, G., Joseph, H., Mouloungui, Z., Bourgeois, P. 2005. Composition of fatty acids triacylglycerols and unsaponifiable matter in *Calophyllum calaba* L. oil from Guadeloupe. *Phytochemistry*. 66, 1825-1831.

Christie, W. W. 1968. Chromatography of the isomeric methylene-interrupted methyl *cis,cis*-octadecadienoates. *J. Chromatogr*. 37, 27-38.

Christie, W. W. 1988. Equivalent chain-lengths of methyl ester derivatives of fatty acids on gas chromatography. *J. Chromatograhy*. 447, 305-314.

Dweck, A. C., Meadows, T. 2002. Tamanu (*Calophyllum inophyllum*): the African, Asian, Polynesian and Pacific *PanaceaTamanu*. *Int. J. Cosmet. Sci*. 24,1-8.

De Greyt, W., Kint, A., Kellens, M., Huyghebaert, A. 1998. Determination of low *trans* levels in refined oils by Fourier transform infrared spectroscopy. *J Am Oil Chem Soc*. 75, 115-118.

Demirbas, A. 2008. *Biodiesel: a realistic fuel alternative for Diesel engines*. Springer, London.

Dutton, H. J. 1979. *Hydrogenation of Fats and Its Significance, in: Geometric and Positional Fatty Acid Isomers.* American Oil Chemists Society, Champaign, Illinois.

Elizabeth V. D., Arumugam, S. 2014. GC-MS analysis of ethanol extract of *Cyperus rotundus* leaves. *International Journal of Current Biotechnology*. 2, 19-23.

El-Mallah, M. H., El-Shami, S. M., Hassanien, M. M. M., Abdel-Razek, A. G. 2011. Effect of chemical refining steps on the minor and major components of cottonseed oil. *Agric. Biol. J. N. Am*. 2, 341-349.

Ergönül, P. G., Köseoˇglu, O. 2014. Changes in α-, β-, γ- and δ-tocopherol contents of mostly consumed vegetable oils during refining process. CyTA - *J. Food*, 12, 199-202.

FAO. 1994. Fats and oils in human nutrition: Report of a Joint FAO/WHO expert consultation. *FAO Food and Nutrition Paper* No. 57. FAO, Rome.

Forestry Department, 2008. Nyamplung *(Callophyllum Inophyllum L.). Sumber Energi Biofuel yang Potensial*, Jakarta, Litbang Kehutanan.

Fellenberg, A. J., Johnson, D. W., Poulus, A., Sharp, P. 1987. Simple mass spectrometric differentiation of the n-3, n-6 and n-9 series of methylene interrupted polyenoic acids. *Biomed. Environ. Mass Spectrom.* 14, 127-130.

Fylaktakidou, K. C., Hadipavlou-Litina, D. J., Litinas, K. E., Nicolaides, D. N., 2004. Natural and synthetic coumarin derivatives with anti-inflammatory/antioxidant activities. *Curr. Pharm.* 10, 3813.

Gibson, R. A. 1988. The effect of diets containing fish and fish oils on disease risk factors in humans. *J. Med.* 18, 713-731.

Grubauer, G., Elias, P. M., Feingold, K. R. 1989. Transepidermal water loss: the signal for recovery of barrier structure and function. *J. Lipid Res.* 30, 323–333.

Gotor, A. A., Rhazi, L. 2016. Effects of refining process on sunflower oil minor components: a review. *OCL.*, 23, D207.

Gui, M. M., Lee, K. T., Bhatia, S. 2008. Feasibility of edible oil vs.non-edible oil vs.waste edible oil as a biodiesel feedstock. *Energy*. 33, 1646–53.

Gunawan, S., Aparamarta, H. W., Kuswandi, K., Widjaja, A., Ju, Y. H. 2014. The utilization of *Xylocarpus moluccensis* seed oil as a biodiesel feedstock in Indonesia. *Ind. Crops Prod.* 52, 286-291.

Gunawan, S., Darmawan, R., Nanda, M., Setiawan, A. D., Fansuri, H. 2013. Proximate composition of *Xylocarpus moluccensis* seeds and their oils. *Ind. Crops Prod.* 41, 107-112.

Gunawan, S., Kasim, N. S., Ju, Y. H. 2008. Separation and purification of squalene from soybean oil deodorizer distillate. *Sep Purif. Technol.* 60, 128-135.

Gunawan, S., Vali, S. R., Ju, Y. H. 2006. Purification and identification of rice bran oil fatty acid steryl and was esters. *J. Am. Oil. Chem. Soc.*, 83, 449.

Hathurusingha, S., Ashwath, N., Midmore, D. 2011. Periodic variation in kernel oil content and fatty acid profiles of *Calophyllum Inophyllum* L.: A potential biodiesel feedstock in Australia, *Biomass Bioenerg.*, 35, 3448-3452.

Hamburger, M. O., Cordell, G. A. 1987. A direct bioautographic TLC assay for compounds possessing antibacterial activity. *J. Nat. Prod.* 50,19-22.

Haugh, A, Høstmark, A. T., Harstad, O. M. 2007. Bovine milk in human nutrition - a review. *Lipids Health Dis.*, 6, 25.

Hejazi, L., Ebrahimi, D., Guilhaus, M., Hibbert, D. B. 2009. Discrimination among geometrical isomers of α–linolenic acid methyl ester using low energy electron ionization mass spectrometry. *J. Am. Soc. Mass. Spectrom.* 20, 1272-1280.

Hemavathy, J., Prabhakar, J. V. 1990. Lipid composition of *Calophyllum inophyllum* kernel. *J Am Oil Chem Soc.* 53, 1578–1579.

Heller, H., Scheafer, M., Schulten, K. 1993. Molecular dynamics simulation of a bilayer of 200 lipids in the gel and in the liquid-crystal phases. *J. Phys. Chem.* 97, 8343–8360.

Hoffmann, G. 1989. *The chemistry and technology of edible oils and fats and their fat products*. Academic, New York, pp139-200.

Holman, R. T., Rahm, J. J. 1971. Analysis and characterization of polyunsaturated fatty acids. *Prog. Chem. Fats Other Lipids*, 9, 15-90 (DOI: 10.1016/0079-6832(71)90024-3).

IUPAC-IUBMB. 1996. Nomenclature of carbohydrates (Recommendations 1996). *Pure Appl. Chem.* 68, 1919-2008.

James, A. T. 1959. Determination of the degree of unsaturation of long chain fatty acids by gas-liquid chromatography. *J. Chromatogr.* 2, 552-561.

Jean M. 2009. *Trees in sustainable farming Auroville, Tamil Nadu* [cited 4 February 2011]; Available from: /http://www.csfbg.org/reports/Trees %20in%20 sustainable%20 farming%20Report.pdfS.

Judd, J. T., Clevidence, B. A., Muesing, R. A., Wittes, J., Sunkin, M.E., Podczasy, J. J. 1994. Dietary *trans* fatty acids: effects of plasma lipids and lipoproteins on healthy men and women. *Am. J. Clin. Nutr.* 59, 861-868.

Kansedo, J., Lee, K. T., Bhatia, S., 2009. *Cerbera odollam* (sea mango) oil as a promising non-edible feedstock for biodiesel production. *Fuel.* 88, 1148-1150.

Karaali, A. 1985. The effects of refining on the chemical composition of Turkish sunflower seed oil. *Eur. J. Lipid Sci. Technol.* 87, 112-117.

Kilham, C., 2004. Tamanu oil. A tropical topical remedy. *Herbal Gram.* 63, 26-31.

Knothe, G. C., Evangelista, S. C., Roque, L. 2009. Cuphea oil as a source of biodiesel with improved fuel properties caused by high content of methyl decan-oatey. *Energ. Fuel,* 23, 1743–7.

Kreps, F., Vrbiková, L., Schmidt, Š. 2014. Influence of industrial physical refining on tocopherol, chlorophyll and beta-carotene content in sunflower and rapeseed oil. *Eur. J. Lipid Sci. Technol*. 116,1572-1582.

Lamer, V. K. 1962. *Retardation of evaporation by monolayers*, Academic Press, New York.

Langstraat, A. 1976. Characteristics and composition of oil-bearing materials. *J. Am. Oil Chem. Soc*. 53, 241-47.

Lee, Y. F., Gibot, A. 1986. *Indigenous edible plants of Sabah*; FRC publication, Sabah Forestry Department: Sandakan, 9.

Lemmens, R. H. M. J. 2003. *Calophyllum* L. In: Lemmens RHMJ, Bunyapraphatsara N (eds) *Plant resources of South-East Asia* no 12(3). Medicinal and poisonous plants 3; Prosea Foundation: Bogor, p 102

Lim, T. K. 2012. *Fruits in Edible medicinal and non-medicinal Plants*; Springer: Netherlands.

Marchand, C. M. 1982. Positional isomers of *trans*-octadecenoic acids in margarine. *Can. I. Food Sc. Tech. J*. 15, 196-199.

Masjuki, H. H. 2010. *Biofuel engine: a new challenge.* Kuala Lumpur, Malaysia: Department of Mechanical Engineering Univerisity of Malaya.

Mohod, A. G., Bhor, P. P., Kadam, Sengar, S. H., Khandetod, Y. P. 2010. Study of properties of *Calophyllum inophyllum* L. Oil and its biodiesel. *Int. J. Agric. Eng*. 3, 125.

McLafferty, F. W. 1959. Molecular rearrangements. *Anal. Chem*. 31, 82-87.

Mjos, S. A., Pettersen, J. 2001. *Improved methods for analysis of fatty acid isomers.* Norwegian Herring Oil and Meal Industry Research Institute, Norway.

Mjos, S. A., Pettersen, J. 2003. Determination of trans double bonds in polyunsaturated fatty acid methyl esters from their electron impact mass spectra. *Eur. J. Lipid Sci. Technol*. 105, 156–164.

Montgomery, D. C. 2005. *Design and analysis of experiments*, 6th Ed.; John Wiley and Sons: New York, 96.

Nergiz, C., Çelikkale, D. 2011. The effect of consecutive steps of refining on squalene content of vegetable oils. *J. Food Sci. Technol.* 48, 382-385.

No SY. 2011. Inedible vegetable oils and their derivatives for alternative diesel fuels in CI engines: a review. *Renew. Sust. Energ. Rev.* 15, 131–49.

Qin, W. H, Lan, H. X., Shan, L. X., Fang, H., Xin, Z. Z., Fen, M. Y. 2007. Gas chromatographic retention time rule and mass spectrometric fragmentation rule of fatty acids and its application in food. *Chin. J. Anal. Chem.* 35, 998-1003.

Ramaraju, A., Ashok, K. T. V. 2011. Biodiesel development from high free fatty acid punnakka oil. *J. Eng. Appl. Sci.* 6, 1–6.

Ribeiro, A., Castro, F., Carvalho, J. 2011. Influence of free fatty acid content in biodiesel production on non-edible oils In Proceeding: *WASTES: Solutions, Treatments, and Opportunities*; European Environment Agency: Portugal.

Roselló, J. Puiggròs, C., Sánchez, J., Chacón, P., Sabín, P., Bou, R., Planas, M. 2009. Evolution of lipid profile, liver function, and pattern of plasma fatty acids according to the type of lipid emulsion administered in parenteral nutrition in the early postoperative period after digestive surgery. *J. Parenter Enteral. Nutr.* 33, 501-12.

Ruggles K. V., Garbarino, J., Liu, Y., Moon, J., Schneider, K., Henneberry, A., Billheimer, J., Millar, J. S., Marchadier, D., Valasek, M. A., Joblin-Mills, A., Gulati, S., Munkacsi, A. B., Repa, J. J., Rader, D., Sturley, S. L. 2013. A functional, genome-wide evaluation of liposensitive yeast identifies the "ARE2 required for viability" (ARV1) gene product as a major component of eukaryotic fatty acid resistance. *J. Biol. Chem.* 289, 4417-31.

Ruiz-Gutierrez, V., Morgado, N., Prada, J. L., Pe´ rez-Jime´nez, F., Muriana, F. J. G. 1998. Composition of Human VLDL Triacylglycerols after Ingestion of Olive Oil and High Oleic Sunflower *Oil. J Nutr*, 128, 570-576.

Santacesaria, E., Vicente, G. M, Di Serio, M., Tesser. 2012. Main technologies in biodiesel production: state of the art and future challenges. *Catal. Today*. 195, 2-13.

Sanford, SD, White, JM, Shah, PS, Wee, C, Valverde, MA, Meier, GR. 2011. *Feedstock and biodiesel characteristics report.*

Sasidharan, S., Chen, Y., Saravanan, D., Sundram, K. M., Latha, L. Y. 2011, Extraction, isolation, and characterization of bioactive compounds from plants' extract. *Afr. J. Tradit. Complement Altern.* Med. 8, 1-10.

Sloan, A. E. 2006. Good for you fats and oils, new nutraceutical opportunities for fats and oils. *Inform.* 17, 68–70.

Shiu, P., Gunawan, S., Hsieh, W. H., Kasim, N. S., Ju, Y. H. 2010. Biodiesel production from rice bran by a two-step in-situ process. *Bioresource Technol.* 101, 984-989.

Sahoo, P. K., Das, L. M., Babu, M. K. G., Naik, S. N. 2007. Biodiesel development from high acid value polanga seed oil and performance evaluation in a CI engine. *Fuel,* 86, 448–54.

Singh, S. P., Singh, D. 2010. Biodiesel production through the use of different sources and characterization of oils and their esters as the substitute of diesel: a review. *Renew. Sust. Energ. Rev.* 14, 200-216.

Sharma, Y. C., Singh, B. 2009. Development of biodiesel: current scenario. *Renew. Sust. Energ. Rev.*, 13, 1646.

SNI 01-3741. 2002. *Indonesian standard of cooking oil*; National Standardization Agency of Indonesia: Jakarta, Indonesia.

Saraf, S., Thomas, B. 2007. Influence of feedstock and process chemistry on biodiesel quality. J Process Safety and Environmental Protection, *Trans. IChemE. Part B*. 85, 360.

Shen, Y. C., Hung, M. C., Wang, L. T., Chen, C. Y. 2003. *Inocalophyllins* A, B and their methyl esters from the seeds of *Calophyllum inophyllum*. *Chem Pharm Bull*. 51, 802-806.

Su, X. H., Zhang, M. L., Li, L. G., Huo, C. H. and Gu, Y. C. 2008. Chemical Constituent of the Plants of the Genus *Calophyllum. Chem Biodivers.* 5, 2579-2608.

Talal, E. M. A. S., Jiang, J., Yuanfa, L. 2013. Chemical refining of sunflower oil: effect on oil stability, total tocopherol, free fatty acids, and color. *Int. J. Eng. Sci. Tech.* 5, 449-454.

Tasan, M., Demirci, M. 2005. Total and individual tocopherol contents of sunflower oil at different steps of refining. *Eur. Food Res. Technol.* 220, 251-254.

Thompson, R. H. 1997. Simplifying fatty acid analyses using a standard set of gas-liquid chromatographic conditions: II. Equivalent chain length values for *cis-* and *trans-* isomers of monoethylenic C18 fatty acid methyl esters for carbowax-20M liquid phase. *J. Chromatographic Sci.* 35, 598-602.

Thoenes, P. 2007. *Biofuels and commodity markets—palm oil focus*. FAO, Commodities and Trade Division. November.

Thiruvengadaravi, K. V., Nandagopal, J., Baskaralingam, P., Sathya Selva Bala, V., Sivanesan, S. 2012. Acid-catalyzed esterification of Karanja (*Pongamia pinnata*) oil with high free fatty acids for biodiesel production. *Fuel,* 98, 1.

Thengane, S. R., Bhosle, S. V., Deodhar, S. R., Pawar, K. D., Kulkarni, D. K., 2006. Micropropagation of Indian laurel (*Calophyllum inophyllum*), a source of anti-HIV compounds. *Curr. Sci. India*, 90, 10.

Umerie, S. C., Okonkwo, I. F., Nwadialor, N. A., Okonkwo, J. C. 2010. Studies on the oil and nutritive value of seeds of *Crotalaria retusa* L. (Fabaceae). *Pakistan J. Nutr*. 9, 912–4.

Uriarte, F. A. J. 2010. *Biofuels from plant oils.* [cited 24 January 2010]; Available from: /http://www.aseanfoundation.org/documents/books/biofuel.pdfS.

Venkanna, B. K, Venkataramana, R. C. 2009. Biodiesel production and optimization from *Calophyllum inophyllum* Linn oil (hone oil)—a three-stage method. *Bioresource Techno*, 100, 5122–5.

Wirawan, S. S. 2008. *Design and construction of biodiesel plant in Indonesia.* [cited 8 February 2011]; Available from: /Http://www.google.com/#hl=en&sugexp=ldymls&xhr=t&q=DESIGNþAND þCONSTRUCTIONþOFþþBIODIESELþPLANTþINþINDONESIA& cp=56&pf=p&sclient=psy&site=&source=hp&aq=f&aqi=&aql=&oq= DESIGNþANDþCONSTRUCTIONþOFþþ BIODIESELþPLANTþINþ INDONESIA&pbx=1&fp=acc969af815715bfS.

Yimdjo, M. C., Azebaze, A. G., Nkengfack, A. E., Meyer, A. M., Bodo, B., Fomum, Z. T., 2004. Antimicrobial and cytotoxic agents from *Calophyllum inophyllum*. *Phytochemistry*. 65, 2789–2795.

Zufarov, O., Schmidt, S., Sekretár, S. 2008. Degumming of rapeseed and sunflower oils. *Acta Chimica Slovaca*. 1, 321-328.

In: Seed Oil
Editor: Nguyen Khanh Dieu Hong
ISBN: 978-1-53613-560-2

Chapter 4

GRAPE SEED OIL: CHEMICAL COMPOSITION, BIOLOGICAL PROPERTIES AND HEALTH BENEFITS

Sana Bellili[1,2], Sabrine Jazi[1,2], Soumaya ben Nasr[1,3], Wissal Dhifi[4], Maria Alcinda Neves[3], Maria da Graça Costa Miguel[3,*] and Wissem Mnif[1,5,†]

[1]Univ. Manouba, ISBST, BVBGR-LR11ES31,
Biotechpole Sidi Thabet, Ariana, Tunisia
[2]Faculty of Sciences of Bizerte, Jarzouna, Bizerte,
University of Carthage, Tunisia

[*] Corresponding author: Dr. Maria da Graça Costa Miguel/ Department of Chemistry and Pharmacy, Laboratory of Chemistry of Natural Products, Faculty of Sciences and Technology, University of Algarve, Gambelas, 8005-139 Faro, Portugal. E-mail: mgmiguel@ualg.pt.

[†] Corresponding author: Dr. Wissem Mnif/ LR11-ES31 Laboratory of Biotechnology and Valorisation of Bio-GeoRessources, Higher Institute of Biotechnology of Sidi Thabet, BiotechPole of Sidi Thabet, 2020, Universiy of Manouba, Tunisia. E-mail: w_mnif@yahoo.fr / Tel: + (216) 98 94 73 71.

[3] Department of Chemistry and Pharmacy, Laboratory of Chemistry of Natural Products, Faculty of Sciences and Technology, University of Algarve, Gambelas, 8005-139 Faro, Portugal
[4] LR17ES03 Physiopathologie, Alimentation et Biomolécules (PAB), Institut Supérieur de Biotechnologie de Sidi Thabet Biotechpole Sidi Thabet, Sidi Thabet, 2020, Université de La Manouba, Tunisie
[5] Faculty of Sciences and Arts in Balgarn PO BOX 60 Balgarn- Sabt Al Olaya 61985, Bisha University, Saudi Arabia

Abstract

During wine production, formation of biomass residue (peel, seed and grape stems) occurs and thus constitute a problem from an environmental point of view. Nevertheless, this residue may be reused with the purpose of obtaining products with beneficial properties for Human beings as well as for the environment. Seeds from grapes can be used in the food industry to obtain oils. This use makes of them a value-added food due to its richness in linoleic acid, vitamin E, and phytosterols responsible for several biological properties such as antioxidant, anti-inflammatory, and anti-hypercholesterolemia activities. In the chapter, the main procedures to obtain grape seed oils, their chemical composition and biological properties will be reviewed.

Keywords: grape seed, oil, chemical composition, antimicrobial activity, antioxidant and anti-inflammatory activities, anticancer activity, cardioprotective activity

Introduction

Vitis vinifera L. (grapes) is a member of the family *Vitaceae*. Grape seeds, grape stems and grape peels (grape pomace) are the waste resulting from the production wine, vinegar and molasses in the wine industry (Yalcin et al., 2017). Almost 30% of wastes are produced in this industry

(Ekici et al., 2014). Dry pomace is constituted by 25% grapes and 20-26% seeds (Yalcin et al., 2017).

For a long time ago, these wastes were burnt, used in composting, for feeding cattle or discarded in open areas, which altogether may negatively affect crop yields and animal production, due to the possible presence of anti-nutritive compounds in pomace grape. Nevertheless, nowadays many approaches have been made for using this waste in several other domains: productions of biodiesel and food industry are only very few examples (García-Lomillo and González-SanJosé, 2017; Fernández et al., 2010; Teixeira et al., 2014).

Alcohol may be produced from the pomace grape, nevertheless, the yield is much higher distilling wine surpluses and this has been the current practice in the European Union (Pardo et al., 2009). According to Shinagawa et al. (2015), the utilization of seeds in the food industry, in contrast to the stems and peels, which are not economically used, may lower the production costs of wine, increasing producer income, because new products may be created for human consumption.

Grape seed extract is mainly constituted by fibers (40%), complex carbohydrates (29%), oil (16%), proteins (11%), and complex phenols (7%) (Felhi et al., 2016). Antioxidant, anti-inflammatory, antimicrobial and anticancer activities are some examples of bioactivities reported for grape seed oil (Garavaglia et al., 2016).

In this chapter, the main procedures to obtain grape seed oils, their chemical composition and biological properties will be briefly reviewed.

CHEMICAL COMPOSITION

Previous to oil extraction, seeds are separated from other grape pomace constituents, including stems and peels, by using mechanical devices (Lavelli et al., 2016).

Grape seed oil (GSO) is traditionally obtained by cold-pressing, including cold screw-pressing, nevertheless other techniques have been described, such as extraction by using organic solvents (petroleum ether, hexane) though Soxhlet extraction or pressurized liquid extraction, supercritical CO_2 extraction, and ultrasound-assisted extraction using non-polar solvents (Pardo et al., 2009; Fernandes et al., 2013; Sabi et al., 2012; da Porto et al., 2013; Lutterodt et al., 2011; Rombaut et al., 2014; 2015; Agostini et al., 2012; Freitas et al., 2013).

Mechanical extraction at room temperature provides a high-quality oil, nevertheless with low yields, due to the mechanical resistance of seeds which are characterized by a woody texture. To increase the yield, mechanical extraction may be done at higher temperatures. The disadvantage in this case is the decrease of oil quality due to the possible degradation of some thermally unstable compounds (Lavelli et al., 2016).

The oil yield is higher using organic solvents (hexane or petroleum ether) residual undesirable traces of these solvents either in health or environmental terms may remain, which are undesirable. In addition, degradations of those compounds that are thermally unstable at boiling point temperatures of those organic solvents may occur (Lavelli et al., 2016).

The supercritical CO_2 extraction of grape seed oil allows obtaining higher yields when compared to the cold pressing process. The supercritical CO_2 extraction of grape seed oil has the advantage over the extraction by solvents of leaving no traces of organic solvents and at the same time, prevents possible degradations of those thermally unstable compounds (Garavaglia et al., 2016; Jokić et al., 2016). In addition, CO_2 used in the supercritical extraction has the advantage to be non-toxic, non-flammable and is relatively cheap. Besides, the separation of CO_2 from the oil, after extraction, is easy to achieve just by depressurizing (Lavelli et al., 2016). Nevertheless, supercritical CO_2 extraction requires an elevated initial investment for acquiring the equipment and technology, which is only profitable if the final product is highly valuable. According to Fiori (2010), such investment is justifiable due to the high demand and market price of grape seed oil.

Several studies have been performed to evaluate the effect of some variables of operating conditions (pressure, temperature, solvent flow and particle size) on the extraction of grape seed oils by supercritical CO_2

extraction (Duba and Fiori, 2015; Pérez et al., 2015; Passos et al., 2010; Fiori et al, 2014; Gómez et al., 1996).

Grape seed oil is constituted by hydrophilic and lipophilic constituents. The majority of biological activities attributed to grape seed oils are due to the hydrophilic constituents (Garavaglia et al., 2016), although the lipophilic vitamin E and essential fatty acids have also an important role in the prevention of some cardiovascular diseases, as neuroprotective, for lowering the cholesterol levels and as antioxidants (Fernandes et al., 2013).

Lipophilic Constituents

The grape seed contains between 6 and 22% of oil: This amount depends on the grape variety as well as the environment conditions during ripening and also on the method of extraction (Beveridge et al., 2005; Akter et al., 2006; Rubio et al., 2009; Tangolar et al., 2009; Pardo et al., 2011; Fiori et al., 2014; Tociu et al., 2017).

Polyunsaturated fatty acids: PUFA (85-90%), mainly linoleic acid (C18:2) (58-78%), predominate in grape seed oils (Shinagawa et al., 2015; Codex Stan 210, 2009). Such as for the oil yield, the variations found in the linoleic acid percentages may also be attributed to the same factors: grape variety (Beveridge et al., 2005; Akter et al., 2006; Tangolar et al., 2009; Ahmadi and Siahsar, 2011; Fernandes et al., 2013; Fiori et al., 2014; Ovcharova et al., 2016; Yalcin et al., 2017); ripening (Rubio et al., 2009); geographical origin (Crews et al., 2006; Fiori et al., 2014); and extraction method (Beveridge et al., 2005; Prado et al., 2012; Pérez et al., 2015). However, Porto et al. (2013) did not find differences in the amounts of the linoleic acid obtained either by ultrasound-assisted extraction or Soxhlet extraction. The authors only reported differences in the amounts of stearic acid. Other factors were also found to be responsible for the variability of linoleic acid percentages in the grape seed oils: time of exposure to gamma irradiation, and microwave heating. In both cases, a higher period of exposure leads to a decrease of the amounts of linoleic acid (Apaydin et al., 2017; Özcan & Al Juhaimi (2017).

Oleic (C18:1) and palmitic acids (C16:0) are also FA with important percentages (12-28% and 5.5-11.0% respectively) in grape seed oils (Codex Stan 210, 2009), whose amounts are also dependent on the same factors reported for linoleic acid (C18: 2) (Akter et al., 2006; Pardo et al., 2009; Rubio et al., 2009; Tangolar et al., 2009; Bada et al., 2015; Ovcharova et al., 2016; Wen et al., 2016; Yalcin et al., 2017). In the cultivar, South Columbia, Akter et al., (2006) found that stearic acid (C18:0) percentage (>15%) was significantly higher than those generally reported for grape seed oils (3.0-6.5%) (Codex Stan 210, 2009).

Tocopherols and tocotrienols are also lipophilic constituents of grape seeds oils. Although α-, β-, γ-, and δ-tocopherol can be found in grape seed oils, tocotrienols (unsaturated forms of tocopherols) are the most abundant, particularly γ-tocotrienol (436 – 1630 mg/kg), followed by α-tocotrienol (56 – 341 mg/kg), depending on the variety of Portuguese grapes (Fernandes et al., 2013). However, other authors (Wen et al., 2016) found higher concentrations of α-tocotrienol (177.77 – 521.11 mg/kg) than γ-tocotrienol (128.87 – 183.70 mg/kg) in several varieties of *V. vinifera* from China. The ratio γ-tocotrienol/α-tocotrienol was >1 in the variety Tempranillo from Toro (Spain), but <1 in the same variety but from Ribera (Spain) (Bada et al., 2015). These results reveal that variety and origin are determinant on the amounts of vitamin E (tocopherols and tocotrienols) in grape seed oils as also reported by several authors (Crews et al., 2006; Shinagawa et al., 2015).

Extraction procedure also influences the amounts of tocopherols and tocotrienols in grape seed oil. Mohamed et al., (2016) reported that supercritical CO_2 extraction of grape seed oil allowed extracting higher amounts of tocopherols and tocotrienols than hexane extraction using the Soxhlet method. Fiori et al., (2014) also reported higher or similar amounts of tocopherols and tocotrienols in grape seed oils obtained by supercritical CO_2 extraction. According to Beveridge et al., (2005), the influence of the extraction method (supercritical CO_2 extraction or petroleum ether extraction) on the total tocopherols and tocotrienols was also dependent on the grape variety.

Phytosterols that constitute the unsaponifiable fraction of oils are also present in grape seed oils. β-Sitosterol is quantitatively the most important phytosterol in grape seed oil, followed by stigmasterol and campesterol (Beveridge et al., 2005; Crews et al., 2006; Pardo et al., 2009; Bada et al., 2015), although the concentrations being highly dependent on the variety and origin. Harvesting period of grapes also affects different amounts of phytosterols according to Rubio et al. (2009). The same authors report that higher total phytosterols could be found in the oils obtained from grapes totally green, that is, before the beginning of ripening (4 weeks after anthesis). The following harvesting periods did not greatly influence the levels of phytosterols, at least as much was found for the first harvesting.

Carotenoids are also present in grape seed oils (Shinagawa et al., 2015; Da Silva and Jorge, 2017), which concentrations varying according to the variety and the extraction method. Supercritical CO_2 procedure allows to extract more carotenoids than solid-liquid extraction (Soxhlet) using hexane (Mohamed et al., 2016).

Volatile compounds were also reported by Bail et al. (2008) in nine diverse grape seeds oils after extraction by solid phase microextraction (SPME) and identification by gas chromatography coupled to mass spectrometry (GC-MS). Organic acids, alcohols, esters, aldehydes and ketones of short carbon chain were detected. The presence or absence of these compounds and their amounts were dependent on grape varieties, seed treatment and oil production conditions. Beyond the presence of caproic acid (hexanoic acid), a typical FA of seed oils, pentanal, hexanal, 2-hexenal, heptanal, trans-2-heptenal and 2-heptanone, 2,3-butandiole, 3-methylbutanol, 2-methylbutanol, hexanol, and ethylhexanoate were also detected in grape seed oils. According to the authors (Bail et al., 2008), the presence of these flavour compounds may result from degradation of fatty acids (e.g., linoleic acid) by oxidation, the activity of enzymes or microbes, processing conditions or even storage conditions. Terpenes were also detected in the volatile fraction, such as α-pinene and limonene (Bail et al., 2008).

Hydrophilic Constituents

Phenols constitute the most important group of hydrophilic compounds of grape seed oils (Garavaglia et al., 2016), nevertheless in relative low amounts (24–53 mg gallic acid equivalent/kg and 28 – 60 mg gallic acid equivalent/kg), when extracted by supercritical CO_2 extraction and solid-liquid extraction by Soxhlet apparatus, respectively. Chinese and Spanish grape seed oil varieties (Wen et al., 2016; Pardo et al., 2009, respectively) had similar concentrations of total phenol of those reported by Garavaglia et al. (2016). The minimal and maximal values reported by the authors (Garavaglia et al., 2016; Mohamed et al., 2016; Wen et al., 2016; Pardo et al., 2009) for each extraction procedure were dependent on the grape varieties used. Two- to twentyfold higher amount of total phenols were detected in several varieties of grape seeds oils by several authors (Bail et al., 2008; Lutterodt et al., 2011), which concentrations were also variety-dependent.

Climate, location, postharvest treatment, gamma irradiation, and storage conditions are other factors that also contribute to the quantitative variability of phenolic compounds in grape seed oils (Lutterodt et al., 2011; Rombaut et al., 2015; Apaydan et al., 2017). Gamma irradiation has a negative effect on the phenol content of grape seed oils, independently of the grape variety (Apaydan et al., 2017). The amounts of these compounds are significantly lower than those detected in sunflower and olive oils (Matthäus, 2008).

The relative low concentrations of phenols in grape seed oil may be attributed to their limited liposolubility, and therefore they remain in the residue (Matthäus, 2008). Phenolic acids (gallic, ferulic, caffeic, vanillin acids), phenolic aldehydes (vanillin), hydroxycinnamic esters (caftaric, coutaric, fertaric acids), monomeric flavanols (catechin, epicatechin and epicatechin-3-*O*-gallate), flavonols and their glucoside derivatives (kampferol, quercetin, quercetin-3-glucoside, quercetin-3-rhamnoside, quercetin-3-galactoside) and diverse oligomer procyanidins (procyanidin B_1, procyanidin B_2) are examples of compounds that may constitute the phenolic fraction of grape seed oils (Matthäus, 2008; Maier et al., 2009; Lutterodt et al., 2011; Agostini et al., 2012; Rombaut et al., 2014; Karaman et al., 2015; Marchi et al., 2015).

BIOLOGICAL PROPERTIES

Many biological properties have been attributed to grape seed oils: antimicrobial, antioxidant, anti-inflammatory, and anti-carcinogenic, antimutagenic, prevention, and delay of cardiovascular diseases, among other activities. However, many of these studies are based on in vitro experiments, in cell cultures or animal models which results may be different from those observed in humans (Garavaglia et al., 2016).

Antimicrobial Activity

The effectiveness of grape seed oils against pathogens depends on the concentration, the microorganism species, including strains level, the pH, and polarity of the matrix (García-Lomillo and González-SanJosé (2017). Whereas several works refer the antimicrobial properties of grape seed oils, other ones did not find any activity, at least for two Gram-positive (*Staphylococcus aureus* ATCC 25923 and *Listeria monocytogenes* ATCC 19118) and two Gram-negative bacteria (*Escherichia coli* O157:H7 ATCC 33150 and *Salmonella enteric* subsp. enteric serovar Typhimurium ATCC 14028) (Karaman et al., 2015). However, other studies showed that grape seed oils had bactericide activity on *Bacillus subtitlis* JN 934392, *E. coli* ATCC 25922 and *S. enteritidis* ATCC 43972, nevertheless, without any activity on *Staphylococcus aureus* ATCC 6538 (Rekik et al., 2016). In the same study, two more oils were assayed: sesame and fenugreek oils. The grape seed oil has better activity than sesame and fenugreek oils. The highest acidity of grape seed oil may partly explain its better antimicrobial activity since fenugreek possessed higher amounts of phenols and the activity was poorer (Rekik et al., 2016). Another study also demonstrated the bactericidal capacity of grape seed oil variety Malvasía against *B.*

cereus, *S. aureus*, *P. aeruginosa* and *E. coli* (Berradre et al., 2016), suggesting the authors that this oil could be used as food additive to combat pathogenic bacteria.

Generally, the antimicrobial activity is attributed to polyphenols and many studies have demonstrated the importance of these secondary metabolites as antimicrobials. These studies were performed using grape seed extracts in which polyphenols predominate (Özcan et al., 2004; Baydar et al., 2006; Sagdic et al., 2011). The studies performed by these authors demonstrated the bactericide activity of grape seed extracts against both spoilage and pathogenic bacteria (*Aeromonas hydrophila*, *Bacillus cereus*, *Enterobacter aerogenes*, *Enterococcus faecalis*, *E. coli*, *E. coli* O157:H7, *Mycobacterium smegmatis*, *Proteus vulgaris*, *Pseudomonas aeruginosa*, *Pseudomonas fluorescens*, *Salmonella enteritidis*, *Salmonella typhimurium*, *S. aureus* and *Yersinia enterocolitica*. The activity against these types of microorganisms has lead to find out the possibility of these extracts to be incorporated into edible coatings with biopolymers (chitosan, gelatin) for preserving and extending shelf-life of fruits and vegetables, not only for their antimicrobial activities, but also for their antioxidant properties (Rubilar et al., 2013; Duran et al., 2016; Shahbazi, 2017).

In conclusion, polyphenols from grape seeds may be considered as good agents for food preservation and as medicine not only for suppressing the growth of pathogenic bacteria but also by preventing oxidation, nevertheless requiring always higher concentrations than the conventional antibiotics, antimicrobials or antioxidants (Yu and Ahmedna, 2013).

Antioxidant and Anti-Inflammatory Activities

PUFA predominate in the grape seed oil. The presence of double bonds in FA triggers oxidation process unless some components being present in the oil can prevent a rapid oxidation. In fact, grape seed oil is relatively stable in oxidative terms which can be explained by the presence not only of the natural lipossoluble antioxidants tocopherols, tocotrienols, carotenoids, chlorophylls but also of the phenols (Pardo et al., 2009;

Mohamed et al., 2016; Hashemi et al., 2017). These compounds are, therefore, important either for the oxidative stability of the grape seed oil itself or can also be a new food ingredient in meat, fish, bakery, dairy products or fruits and vegetables, as natural antioxidants, particularly grape seed extracts in which phenols predominate (Peng et al., 2010; Mielnik et al., 2006; Yerlikaya and Gokoglu, 2010; Ferreira et al., 2014; da Silva et al., 2015; Pateiro et al., 2015; Lavelli et al., 2016 and references therein, Shahbazi, 2017).

The antioxidant activity revealed to be dependent on the variety of grapes (Pardo et al., 2009; Mandic et al., 2008; Yemis et al., 2008), solvent and temperature for extracting grape seed phenols (Chung et al., 2005; Bucić-Kojić et al., 2009), previous treatment of grape seeds (heating) (Kim et al., 2006), some treatments made on grape seed oils, such as γ irradiation for killing harmful bacteria and other microorganisms, or microwave may decrease phenol content and, therefore, the antioxidant capacity of grape seeds oils (Apaydin et al., 2017; Hashemi et al., 2017), or thermal treatment of grape seed extracts (pasteurisation, cooking, baking and sterilisation) (Davidov-Pardo et al., 2011).

Several *in vitro* studies have demonstrated the antioxidant capacity of grape seed extracts for scavenging free radicals such as 2,2'-Azino-di-[3-ethylbenzthiaoline sulphonate (ABTS), 2,2-diphenyl-1-picrylhydrazyl (DPPH) , superoxide anion radicals, peroxyl radicals through the oxygen radical absorbance capacity (ORAC), peroxynitrite among other radicals, or using other methods such as the Ferric Reducing Antioxidant Power (FRAP), chelating activity, the β-carotene-linoleate model system and linoleic acid peroxidation method, oil/oxidative stability index using the Rancimat instrument, peroxide value, conjugated diene value, carbonyl value (Bail et al., 2008; Jokić et al., 2016; Pardo et al., 2009; Shafiee et al., 2003; Ferreira et al., 2014; Wen et al., 2016, Hashemi et al., 2017; Wang et al., 2010; Cádiz-Gurrea et al., 2017).

The capacity for scavenging superoxide anion radicals was already reported (Yamaguchi et al., 1999) using a spin-trapping electron spin resonance (ESR) method. They found that when the degree of polymerization of procyanidins present in grape seed extracts was higher, the superoxide anion radicals scavenging activity was stronger. In addition, the activity was also better when grape seed extracts were combined with α-tocopherol (Yamaguchi et al., 1999). The degree of procyanidins' polymerization on the antioxidant activity measured through diverse methods (FRAP, ORAC, ABTS) was also reported recently by Cádiz-Gurrea et al., (2017) when compared the activity results of grape seed extracts with those of cocoa. Higher content of the oligomeric forms of flavan-3-ols, along with higher content of gallic acid in the grape seed extracts than in cocoa extracts resulted in better capacity for scavenging the peroxyl and ABTS free radicals (Cádiz-Gurrea et al., 2017). According to Guendez et al., (2005), the free radical scavenging activity of nine grape seed extracts obtained from several Hellenic varieties of *V. vinifera* and cultivated in Greece correlated strongly with procyanidin B1, despite its relative low amount in the whole polyphenol content.

Beyond the direct action of phenols of grape seed extracts on free radicals, scavenging them, the same compounds may also act at the gene expression levels and production of some antioxidant enzymes, such as glutathione peroxidase (GPx), catalase (CAT) and superoxide dismutase (SOD), avoiding tissue damages induced by oxidative stress. Yang et al. (2014) reported that grape seed extracts increased the mRNA expression levels and activities of CAT and SOD in primary muscle cells (PMC), isolated from the gluteal muscles of a local breed, south China, when previously treated with hydrogen peroxide.

The antioxidant capacity of the phenols' extracts may also be directed towards human health. Due to the capacity for scavenging free radicals, grape seed extracts are marketed as a dietary health supplement (Yen et al., 2015). According to many authors, the antiproliferative effect of grape seed extracts against several cancer cell lines (human bladder, colorectal, breast, oral) involves several mechanisms including apoptosis, DNA damage and oxidative stress (Stankovic et al., 2008; Raina et al., 2013; Dinicola et al., 2014; Yen et al., 2015).

The vasodilation properties of procyanidins, important on the regulation of vascular homeostasis, seem to be attributed to their antioxidant properties (Ahmad et al., 2013). The antioxidant activity, due to the presence of procyanidins of grape seed extracts along with tannins, was also reported by Shafiee et al. (2003). Those extracts were able to protect LDL (low-density lipoproteins) from oxidation in the presence of the generating peroxynitrite anion (ONNO-) 3-morpholinosydnonimine molecule (SIN-1) as well as impair the production of superoxide anion radical by THP-1 cells (Shafiee et al., 2003). The importance of preventing LDL oxidation is the fact that oxidized LDL is involved in the early inflammation and further in more advanced phases, in the atherosclerotic lesions. For this reason, procyanidins-rich grape seed extract may retard the development of atherosclerotic lesions reducing LDL oxidation (Shafiee et al., 2003).

The anti-inflammatory activity of grape seed extracts was also reported by Cádiz-Gurrea et al. (2017). The authors found that those extracts, at concentrations higher than 60 mg/mL, decrease the mRNA expression of monocyte chemoattractant protein-1 (MCP-1) (a pro-inflammatory cytokine) in human umbilical vein endothelial (HUVEC) cells.

As reported above, procyanidins of grape seed extracts are able to scavenge free radicals, to prevent lipid peroxidation and to inhibit the formation of pro-inflammatory cytokines, they possess, therefore, anti-inflammatory activity (Georgiev et al., 2014). The administration of procyanidins, extracted from grape seeds, to rats with arthritis induced by carrageenan lowered the content of nitric oxide (NO), interleukin-1β (IL-1β), tumour necrosis factor α (TNF- α) and prostaglanin E2 (PGE2) in the exsudate of edema paws (Li et al., 2001). *In vitro* studies also reported that grape seed extracts inhibited the overproduction of NO and PGE2, suppressed the inducible nitric oxide synthase expression, and inhibited the translocation of nuclear factor κB (NF-κB) to nucleus in endotoxin-stimulated RAW 264.7 macrophages (Terra et al., 2007). In addition, grape seed extracts may also increase the levels of the anti-inflammatory cytokines IL-2 and IL-4 in the colonic tissues. All of these facts inhibit inflammatory cell infiltration and oxidative damage in those tissues (Wang et al., 2010a, Wang et al., 2010b; Li et al., 2008).

Anti-Cancer or Anti-Tumor Activity

A large number of chemical components from fruits and vegetables (phytochemicals) have been reported to be protective against the initiation, promotion and/or progression of experimental chemical carcinogenesis (Wattenberg et al., 1996). The field of cancer chemoprevention has emerged in which natural and synthetic compounds have been examined for their capacity to reverse, inhibit or delay the cancer process (Stoner and Mukhtar, 1995).

One group of promising chemopreventive phytochemicals is the proanthocyanidins which are very present in grape seeds of *Vitis vinifera* cultivars (Fuleki and Ricardo, 1997). A number of studies have demonstrated that proanthocyanidins extracted from various natural products are effective inhibitors of carcinogenesis in several animal models (Mukhtar et al., 1994; Castonguay et al., 1997).

Bomser et al. (1999) studied the anti-tumor promoting activity of a polyphenolic fraction from grape seeds (GSP) was examined in CD-1 mouse skin epidermis. They evaluated the ability of this fraction to inhibit 12-O-tetradecanoylphorbol-13-acetate (TPA)-induced tumor promotion. Their data suggested that polyphenolic extract from grape seed has the potential to be an effective chemopreventative agent towards mouse skin tumorigenesis and possibly other tumor models as well.

Kim et al. (2004) demonstrated that grape seed extract (GSE) is chemopreventive in an animal model of breast cancer. It has been reported that this complex inhibited the growth of cancer cells in cell culture (Agarwal et al., 2000; Sharma et al., 2004).

Grape seed proanthocyanidins were also reported as being possible chemopreventive agents for colon cancer by inhibiting the expression of both vascular endothelial growth factor (VEGF) and angiopoietin 1 (Ang1), through reducing reactive oxygen species in human colon cancer SW620 cells (Huang et al., 2012). According to the authors, they can be considered as effective antiangiogenic agents. Procyanidins from grape seed extracts were able to inhibit the growth of colon cancer cells (CaCo2 cells) and increased the apoptosis (Engelbrecht et al., 2007), but did not affect the normal colon cell line (NCM460). The increased apoptosis observed in the treated cells could be attributed to the attenuation of the phosphoinositide 3-kinase (PI3-kinase) (p110 and p85 subunits) and decreased protein kinase B (PKB) Ser473 phosphorylation (Engelbrecht et al, 2007).

The synthesis of empty lipid nanocarriers, such as grape seed oil and other natural oils, with antioxidant and antitumor effectiveness against two tumour cells [human breast adenocarcinoma (MDA-MB 231) and epitheloid cervix carcinoma (HeLa)] was reported by Lacatusu et al. (2015). According to the authors, such study reveals the potentiality of natural lipid nanocarriers, without the presence of synthetic drugs, as bioactive products. In addition, if associated with anticancer drugs, the lipid nanocarriers may improve the therapeutic efficacy of these drugs (Lacatusu et al., 2015).

Anti-Hypercholesterolemic and Cardioprotactor Effects

The generation of free radicals may specifically affect the myocardium because of the low antioxidant defense systems in cardiac tissue (Odom et al., 1992). GSO fights free radicals and increased the antioxidant capacity of the blood. It improves endothelial function (elasticity or ability of the blood vessel wall to expand and contract). Hypertriglyceridemia is a powerful predictor of atherogenic cardiovascular diseases. Several studies reported the remarkable effect of grape seed extracts on the regulation of dyslipidemia and cholesterolaemia, particularly proanthocyanins (Quesada et al, 2009; Mildner-Szkudlarz and Bajerska, 2013).

Hypercholesterolemia is a risk factor for cardiovascular disease, including atherosclerosis (Madamanchi et al., 2005). Control of hyperlipidaemia was verified with grape seed oil (GSO) consumption (Vijaimohan et al., 2006; Gorinstein et al., 2003; Baba et al., 1999) and it has been shown that supplementation with the oil significantly reduced triglycerides and LDL-cholesterol level in rats treated by fat diets.

From the nutritional and therapeutic point of view, grape seed oil (GSO) has a high linoleic acid content (important for prostaglandin synthesis, which has an influence on platelet aggregation and inflammatory processes), high vitamin E content (helps to reduce the risk of suffering arteriosclerosis) and low values of cholesterol and therefore recognized as beneficial to prevent heart and circulation problems (Oomah et al., 1998; Martinez et al., 1986; Sineiro et al., 1995; Badaa et al., 2015).

Linoleic acid (LA) is associated with promotion of cardiovascular health by down-regulating low-density lipoprotein cholesterol (LDL-c) production (Kim et al., 2010). Vivancos and Moreno (2008) observed β-sitosterol (phytosterol largely found in GSO) may prevent the release of pro-inflammatory mediators by oxidized low-density lipoprotein-stimulated (oxLDL) macrophage on oxidative stress and eicosanoid synthesis.

As known, GSO composition is based on linoleic acid (LA), and others bioactive compound such as phytosterols. Numerous sources in the literature pointed to phytosterols role in cholesterol absorption reduction in the intestine and, consequently, a decrease in plasma cholesterol levels. The plant sterols were demonstrated to be able to lower blood cholesterol by inhibiting cholesterol absorption (Abuajah et al., 2015). According to Nash (2004), GSO consumption of up to 45 grams of oil per day demonstrated increased HDL-cholesterol and reduced LDL-cholesterol levels in respectively 13 and 7% patients.

Shinagawa et al. (2015) studied the effect of chronic consumption of GSO, obtained from the Brazilian market, in biochemical markers and inflammation of healthy rats. They demonstrated that GSO consumption did not induce significant metabolic changes, however, the contribution to an increase in the levels of HDL was suggested even a rise in levels of serum lipid peroxidation was noticed.

REFERENCES

Abuajah CI, Ogbonna AC, Osuji CM (2015) Functional components and medicinal properties of food: a review. *J Food Sci Technol.* 52(5):2522-9. doi: 10.1007/s13197-014-1396-5.

Agarwal C, Sharma Y, Zhao J, Agarwal R (2000) A polyphenolic fraction from grape seeds causes irreversible growth inhibition of breast carcinoma MDA-MB468 cells by inhibiting mitogen-activated protein kinases activation and inducing G1 arrest and differentiation. *Clin. Cancer Res.* 6: 2921–2930.

Agostini F, Bertussi RA, Agostini G, dos Santos ACA, Rossato M, Vanderlinde R (2012) Supercrital extraction from vinification residues: fatty acids, α-tocopherol, and phenolic compounds in the oil seeds from different varieties of grape. *The Scientific World Journal*, Volume 2012, Article ID 790486, 9 pages doi:10.1100/2012/790486.

Ahmad A, Khan RMA, Alkharfy KM (2013) Effects of selected bioactive natural products on the vascular endothelium. *Journal of Cardiovascular Pharmacology*, 62: 111-121.

Ahmadi SM, Siahsar BA (2011) Analogy of physicochemical attributes of two grape seeds cultivars. *Ciencia e Investigación Agraria*, 38: 291-301.

Akter H, Hamid S, Bashir R (2006) Variation in lipid composition and physico-chemical constituent among six cultivars of grape seed. *Journal of the Chemical Society of Pakistan*, 28: 97-100.

Apaydin D, Demirci AS, Gecgel U (2017) Effect of gamma irradiation on biochemical properties of grape seeds. *Journal of the American Oil Chemistry's Society*, 94: 57-67.

Baba NH, Antoniades K, Habbal Z (1999) Effects of dietary canola, olive, and linolenic acid enriched olive oils on plasma lipids, lipid peroxidation, and lipoprotein lipase activity in rats. *Nutr Res.* 19(4), 601-612.

Bada JC, León-Camacho M, Copovi P, Alonso L (2015) Characterization of grape seed oil from wines with protected denomination of origin

(PDO) from Spain. *Grasas y Aceites*, 66: http://dx.doi.org/10.3989/gya.1063142.

Bail S, Stuebiger G, Krist S, Unterweger H, Buchbauer G (2008) Characteristics of various grape seed oils by volatile compounds, triacylglycerol composition, total phenols and antioxidant capacity. *Food Chemistry*, 108: 1122–1132.

Baydar NG, Sagdic O, Özcan G, Cetin S (2016) Determination of antibacterial effects and total phenolic contents of grape (*Vitis vinifera* L.) seed extracts. *International Journal of Food Science and Technology*, 41: 799-804.

Berradre M, Vides A, de Rodriguéz GO, Soto L, Sulbarán B, Fernández V, Peña J (2016) Physicochemical characterization and antibacterial activity of grape seed oil (*Vitis vinifera*) variety Malvasía. *Revista de la Facultad de Agronomia (LUZ)*, 33: 39-58.

Beveridge THY, Girard B, Kopp T, Drover JCG (2005) Yield and composition of grape seed oils extracted by supercritical carbon dioxide and petroleum ether: varietal effects. *Journal of Agricultural and Food Chemistry*, 53: 1799-1804.

Bomser JA, Singletary KW, Wallig MA, Smith MA (1999) Inhibition of TPA-induced tumor promotion in CD-1 mouse epidermis by a polyphenolic fraction from grape seeds. *Cancer Lett*. 135:151-157.

Bucić-Kojić A, Planinić M, Tomas S, Jakobek L, Seruga M (2009) Influence of solvent and temperature on extraction of phenolic compounds from grape seed, antioxidant activity and colour of extract. *International Journal of Food Science and Technology*, 44: 2394-2401.

Cádiz-Gurrea ML, Borrás-Linares I, Lozano-Sanchez J, Joven J, Fernández-Arroyo S, Segura-Carretero A (2017) Cocoa and grape seed byproducts as a source of antioxidant and anti-inflammatory proanthocyanidins. *International Journal of Molecular Sciences*, 18: 376, doi:10.3390/ijms18020376.

Castonguay A, Gali HU, Perchellet EM, GAo XM, Boukharta M, Jalbert G, Okuda T, Yoshida T, Hatano T, Perchellet JP (1997) Antitumorigenic and antipromoting activitiesof ellagic acid, ellagitannins and oligomeric anthocyanin and procyanidin. *Int. J. Oncol*. 10: 367-373.

Chung HK, Choi CS, Park WJ, Kang MH (2005) Radical scavenging activity of grape-seed extracts prepared from different solvents. *Food Science and Biotechnology*, 14: 715-721.

Codex Stan 210, 2009. Codex Standard for Named Vegetable Oils. *Codex-Stan* 210-1999, pp. 1–13.

Crews C, Hough P, Godward J, Brereton P, Lees M, Guiet S, Winkelmann W (2006) Quantitation of the main constituents of some authentic grape-seed oils of different origin. *Journal of Agricultural and Food Chemistry*, 54: 6261-6265.

Da Porto C, Porretto E, Decorti D (2013) Comparison of ultrasound-assisted extraction with conventional extraction methods of oil and polyphenols from grape (*Vitis vinifera* L.) seeds. *Ultrasonics Sonochemistry*, 20: 1076-1080.

da Silva AC, Jorge N (2017) Bioactive compounds of oils extracted from fruits seeds obtained from agroindustrial waste. *European Journal of Lipid Science and Technology*, 119: DOI: 10.1002/ejlt.201600024.

da Silva DF, Matumoto-Pintro PT, Bazinet L, Couillard C, Britten M (2015) Effect of commercial grape extracts on the cheese-making properties of milk. *Journal of Dairy Science*, 98: 1552-1562.

Davidov-Pardo G, Arozarena I, Marín-Arroyo MR (2011) Stability of polyphenolic extracts from grape seeds after thermal treatments. *European Food Research and Technology*, 232: 211-220.

Dinicola S, Pasqualato A, Cucina A, Coluccia P, Ferranti F, Canipari R, Catizone A, Proietti S, d'Anselmi F, Ricci G, Palombo A, Bizzarri M (2014) Grape seed extract suppresses MDA-MB231 breast cancer cell migration and invasion. *European Journal of Nutrition*, 53: 421-431.

Duba KS, Fiori L (2015) Supercritical CO_2 extraction of grape seed oil: effects of process parameters on the extraction kinetics. *The Journal of Supercritical Fluids*, 98: 33-43.

Duran M, Aday MS, Zorba NND, Temizkan R, Büyükcan MB, Caner C (2016) Potential of antimicrobial active packaging 'containing natamycin, nisin, pomegranate and grape seed extract in chitosan coating' to extend shelf life of fresh strawberry. *Food and Bioproducts Processing*, 98: 354-363.

Ekici L, Simsek Z, Ozturk I, Sagdic O, Yetim H (2014) Effects of temperature, time, and pH on the stability of anthocyanin extracts: prediction of total anthocyanin content using nonlinear models. *Food Analytical Methods*, 7: 1328-1336.

Engelbrecht AM, Mattheyse M, Ellis B, Loos B, Thomas M, Smith R, Peters S, Smith C, Myburgh K (2007) Proanthocyanidin from grape seeds inactivates the PI3-kinase/PKB pathway and induces apoptosis in a colon cancer cell line. *Cancer Lett*ers, 258: 144–153.

Felhi S, Baccouchi N, Salah HB, Smaoui S, Allouche N, Gharsallah N, Kadri A (2016) Nutritional constituents, phytochemical profiles, in vitro antioxidant and antimicrobial properties, and gas chromate-graphy-mass spectrometry analysis of various solvent extracts from grape seeds *(Vitis vinifera* L.) *Food Science and Biotechnology*, 25: 1537-1544.

Fernandes L, Casal S, Cruz R, Pereira JA, Ramalhosa E (2013) Seed oil often traditional Portuguese grape varieties with interesting chemical and antioxidant properties. *Food Research International*, 50: 161-166.

Fernández CM, Ramos MJ, Pérez A, Rodríguez JF (2010) Production of biodiesel from winery waste: extraction, refining and trances-terification of grape seed oil. *Bioresource Technology*, 101: 7019-7024.

Ferreira AS, Nunes S, Castro A, Ferreira P, Coimbra MA (2014) Influence of grape pomace extract incorporation on chitosan films properties. *Carbohydrate Polymers*, 113: 490-499.

Fiori L (2010) Supercritical extraction of grape seed oil at industrial-scale: plant and process design, modeling, economic feasibility. *Chemical Engineering and Processing: Process Intensification*, 49: 866-872.

Fiori L, Lavelli V, Duba KS, Harsha PSC, Mohamed HB, Guella G (2014) Supercritical CO_2 extraction of oil from seeds of six grape cultivars: modelling of mass transfer kinetics and evaluation of lipid profiles and tocol contents. *The Journal of Supercritical Fluids*, 94: 71-80.

Freitas LS, Dariva C, Jacques RA, Caramão EB (2013) Effect of experimental parameters in the pressurized liquid extraction of Brazilian grape peel oil. *Separation and Purification Technology*, 116: 313-318.

Fuleki T, Ricardo da Silva JM (1997) Catechin and Procyanidin Composition of Seeds from Grape Cultivars Grown in Ontario. *J. Agric. Food Chem.* 45: 1156-1160.

Garavaglia J, Merkoski MM, Oliveira A, Marcadenti A (2016) Grape seed oil compounds: biological and chemical actions for health. *Nutrition and Metabolic Insights*, 9: 59-64.

García-Lomillo J, González-SanJosé ML (2017) Applications of wine pomace in the food industry: approaches and functions: *Comprehensive Reviews in Food Science and Food Safety*, 16: 3-22.

Georgiev V, Anamga A, Tsolova V (2014) Recent advances and uses of grape flavonoids as nutraceuticals. *Nutrients*, 6: 391-415.

Gómez AM, López CP, de la Ossa EM (1996) Recovery of grape seed oil by liquid and supercritical carbon dioxide extraction: a comparison with conventional solvent extraction. *The Chemical Engineering Journal*, 61: 227-231.

Gorinstein S, Leontowicz H, Leontowicz M, Lojek A, Číž M, Krzeminski R, Zachwieja Z, Jastrzebski Z, Delgado-Licon E, Martin-Belloso O, Trakhtenberg S (2003) Seed oil improve lipid metabolism and increase antioxidant potential in rats fed diets containing cholesterol. *Nutr Res.* 23(3), 317-330.

Guendez R, Kallithrapa S, makris DP, Kefalas P (2005) Determination of low molecular weight polyphenolic constituents in grape (*Vitis vinifera* sp.) seed extracts: correlation with antiradical activity. *Food Chemistry*, 89: 1-9.

Hashemi SMB, khaneghah AM, Nikmaram N, raesi S, Rahman MS, Avallone S (2017) Heating, microwave and UV irradiation effects on oxidative stability of Sardasht red grape (*Vitis vinifera* cultiv. Sardasht) seed oil. *International Journal of Food Science and Technology*, 52: 1341-1347.

Huang S, Yang N, Liu Y, Gao J, Huang T, Hu L, Zhao J, Li Y, Li C, Zhang X (2012) Grape seed proanthocyanidins inhibit colon cancer-induced angiogenesis through suppressing the expression of VEGF and Ang1. *International Journal of Molecular Medicine,* 30: 1410–1416.

Jayaprakasha GK, Singh RP, Sakariah KK (2001) Antioxidant activity of grape seed (*Vitis vinifera*) extracts on peroxidation models *in vitro*. *Food Chemistry*, 73: 285-290.

Jokić S, Bijuk M, Aladić K, Bilić M, Molnar M (2016) Optimisation of supercritical CO_2 extraction of grape seed oil using response surface methodology. *International Journal of Food Science and Technology*, 51: 403-410.

Karaman S, Karasu S, Tornuk F, Toker OS, Geçgel Ü, Sagdic O, Özcan N, Gül O (2015) Recovery potential of cold press byproducts obtained from the edible oil industry: physicochemical, bioactive and antimicrobial properties. *Journal of Agricultural and Food Chemistry*, 63: 2305-2313.

Kim D J, Jeon G, Sung J, Oh SK, Hong HC, Lee J (2010) Effect of grape seed oil supplementation on plasma lipid profile in rats. *Food Science and Biotechnology*. 19(1): 249-252. http://dx.doi. org/10.1007/s10068-010-0035-9.

Kim S-Y, Jeong S-M, Park W-P, Nam KC, Ahn DU, Lee S-C (2006) Effect of heating conditions of seeds on the antioxidant activity of grape seed extracts. *Food Chemistry*, 97: 472-479.

Lacatusu I, Badea N, Badea G, Loos J, Huang T, Hu L, Zhao J, Li Y, Li C, Zhang X (2015) Lipid nanocarriers based on natural oils with high activity against oxygen free radicals and tumor cell proliferation. *Materials Science and Engineering: C Materials for Biological Applications,*56: 88–94.

Lavelli V, Torri L, Zeppa G, Fiori L, Spigno G (2016) Recovery of wine making by-products for innovative food applications. *Italian Journal of Food Science*, 28: 542-564.

Li WG, Zhang XY, Wu YJ, Tian X (2001) Anti-inflammatory effect and mechanism of proanthocyanidins from grape seeds. *Acta Pharmacologica Sinica*, 22: 1117-1120.

Li XL, Cai YQ, Qin H, Wu YJ (2008) Therapeutic effect and mechanism of proanthocyanidins from grape seeds in rats with TNBS-induced ulcerative colitis. *Canadian Journal of Physiology and Pharmacology*, 86: 841-849.

Lutterodr H, Slavin M, Whent M, Turner E, Yu LL (2011) Fatty acid composition, oxidative stability, antioxidant and antiproliferative properties of selected cold-pressed grape seeds oils and flours. *Food Chemistry*, 128: 391-399.

Madamanchi NR, Vendrov A, Runge MS (2005) Oxidative Stress and Vascular Disease. *Arterioscler Thromb Vasc Biol*. 25(1): 29-38.

Maier T, Schieber A, Kammerer DR, Carle R (2009) Residues of grape (*Vitis vinifera* L.) seed oil production as a valuable source of phenolic antioxidants. *Food Chemistry*, 112: 551-559.

Mandic AI, Dilas SM, Ćetković GS, Čanadanović-Brunet JM, Tumbas VT (2008) Polyphenolic composition and antioxidant activities of grape seed extract. *International Journal of Food Properties*, 11: 713-726.

Marci F, Seraglia R, Molin L, traldi P, de Rosso M, Panighel A, della Vedova A, Gardiman M, Giust M, Carraro R, Flamimi R (2015) Characterization of seed proanthocyanidins of thirty-two red and white hybrid grape varieties. *Vitis*, 54: 121-128.

Martinez Massanet G, Montiel JA, Pando E, Rodriguez LF (1986) Study of agricultural by-products. II. Fatty acid composition of Palomino grapeseed oil. *Grasas Aceites*. 37: 233-236.

Matthäus B (2008) Virgin grape seed oil: is it really a nutritional highlight? *European Journal of Lipid Science and Technology*, 110: 645-650.

Mielnik MB, Olsen E, Vogt G, Adeline D, Skrede G (2006) grape seed extract as antioxidant in cooked, cold stored turkey meat. *LWT - Food Science and Technology*, 39: 191-198.

Mildner-Szkudlarz S, Bajerska J (2013) Protective effect of grape by-product-fortified breads against cholesterol/colic acid diet-induced hypercholesterolaemia in rats. *Journal of the Science of Food and Agriculture*, 93: 3271-3278.

Mohamed HB, Duba KS, Fiori L, Abdelgawed H, Tlili I, Tounekti T, Zrig A (2016) Bioactive compounds and antioxidant activities of different grape (Vitis vinifera L.) seed oils extracted by supercritical CO_2 and organic solvent. *LWT – Food Science and Technology*, 74: 557-562.

Mukhtar H, Katiyar SK, Agarwal R. (1994). Green tea and skin anticarcinogenic effects. *J Invest Dermatol*. 102:3-7

Nash DT (2004) Cardiovascular risk beyond LDL-C levels. Other lipids are performers in cholesterol story. *Postgrad Med*. 116(3):11–15.

Odom AL, Hatwig CA, Stanley JS, Benson AM (1992) Biochemical determinants of Adriamycin toxicity in mouse liver, heart and intestine. *Biochem Pharmacol*. 43: 831–836.

Oomah BD, Liang J, Godfrey D, Mazza G (1998) Microwave, heating of grapeseed: Effect on oil quality. *J. Agric. Food Chem*. 46: 4017-4021.

Ovcharova T, Zlatanov T, Zhatanov M, Dimitrova R (2016) Chemical composition of seeds of four Bulgarian grape varieties. *Ciência e Técnica Vitivinícola*, 31: 31-40.

Özcan MM, Al Juhaimi FY (2017) Effect of microwave roasting on yield and fatty acid composition of grape seed oil. *Chemistry of Natural Compounds*, 53: DOI 10.1007/s10600-017-1926-2.

Özkan G, Sagdic O, Baydar NG, Kurumahmutoglu Z (2004) Antibacterial activities and total phenolic contents of grape pomace extracts. *Journal of the Science of Food and Agriculture*, 84: 1807–1811.

Pardo JE, Fernández E, Rubio M, Alvarruiz A, Alonso GL (2009) Characterization of grape seed oil from different grape varieties. *European Journal of Lipid Science and Technology*, 111: 188-193.

Pardo JE, Rubio M, Pardo A, Zied DC, Alvarez-Ortí M (2011) Improving the quality of grape seed oil by maceration with grinded fresh grape seeds. *European Journal of Lipid Science Tehnology*, 113: 1266-1272.

Passos CP, Silva RM, da Silva FA, Coimbra MA, Silva CM (2010) Supercritical fluid extraction of grape seed (*Vitis vinifera* L.) oil. Effect of the operating conditions upon oil composition and antioxidant capacity. *Chemical Engineering Journal*, 160: 634-640.

Pateiro M, Lorenzo JM, Vázquez JA, franco D (2015) oxidation stability of pig liver pâté with increasing levels of natural antioxidants (grape and tea). *Antioxidants*, 4: 102-123.

Peng X, Ma Y, Cheng K-W, Jiang Y, Chen F, Wang M (2010) The effects of grape seed extract fortification on the antioxidant activity and quality attributes of bread. *Food Chemistry*, 119: 49-53.

Pérez C, del Castillo MLR, Gil C, Blanch GP, Flores G (2015) Supercritical fluid extraction of grape seeds: extract chemical composition, antioxidant activity and inhibition of nitrite production in LPS – stimulated Raw 264.7 cells. *Food and Function*, DOI: 10.1039/c5fo00325c.

Porto C, Porretto E, Decorti D (2013) Comparison of ultrasound-assisted extraction with conventional extraction methods of oil and polyphenols from grape (Vitis vinifera L.) seeds. *Ultrasonics Sonochemistry*, 20: 1076-1080.

Prado JM, Dalmolin I, Carareto NDD, Basso RC, Meirelles AJA, Oliveira JV, Batista EAC, Meireles MAA (2012) Supercritical fluid extraction of grape seed: process scale-up, extarc chemical composition and economic evaluation. *Journal of Food Engineering*, 109: 249-257.

Quesada H, del Bas JM, Pajuelo D, Díaz S, Fernandez-Larrea J, Pinent M, Arola L, Saladó MJ, Bladé C (2009) Grape seed proanthocyanidins correct dyslipidemia assocaited with a high-fat diet in rats and repress genes controlling lipogenesis and VLDL assembling in liver. *International Journal of Obesity*, 33: 1007-1012.

Raina K, Tyagi A, Kumar D, Agarwal R, Agarwal C (2013) Role of oxidative stress in cytotoxicity of grape seed extract in human bladder cancer cells. *Food and Chemical Toxicology*, 61: 187-195.

Rekik DM, Khedir SB, Moalla KK, Kammoun NG, Rebai T, Sahmoun Z (2016) Evaluation of wound healing properties of grape seed, sesame, and fenugrrek oils. *Evidence-Based Complementary and Alternative Medicine*, Article ID 7965689, http://dx.doi.org/10.1155/2016/7965689.

Rombaut N, Savoire R, Thomasset B, Bélliard T, Castello J, van Hecke E, Lanoisellé J-L (2014) Grape seed extraction: interest of supercritical fluid extraction and gas-assisted mechanical extraction for enhancing polyphenol co-extraction in oil. *Comptes Rendus Chimie*, 17: 284-292.

Rombaut N, Savoire R, Thomasset B, Castello J, van Hecke E, Lanoisellé J-L (2015) Optimization oil yield and oil total phenolic content during grape seed cold screw pressing. *Industrial Crops and Products*, 63: 26-33.

Rubilar JF, Cruz RMS, Silva HD, Vicente AA, Khmelinskii I, Vieira MC (2013) Physico-mechanical properties of chitosan films with carvacrol and grape seed extract. *Journal of Food Engineering*, 115: 466-474.

Rubio M, alvarez-Ortí M, Alvarruiz A, Fernández E, Pardo JE (2009) Characterization of oil obtained from grape seeds colected during berry development. *Journal of Agricultural and Food Chemistry*, 57: 2812-2815.

Sabir A, Unver A, Kara Z (2012) The fatty acid and tocopherol constituents of the seed oil extracted from 21 grape varieties *(Vitis* spp.). *Journal of the Science of Food and Agriculture*, 92: 1982-1987.

Sagdic O, Ozturk I, Yilmaz MT, Yetim H (2011) Effect of grape pomace extracts obtained from different grape varieties on microbial quality of beef patty. *Journal of Food Science*, 76: M515–M521.

Shafiee M, Carbonneau MA, Urban N, Descomps B, Leger CL (2003) Grape and grape seed extract capacities at protecting LDL against oxidation generated by Cu2+, AAPH or SIN-1 and at decreasing superoxide THP-1 cell production. A comparison to other extracts or compounds. *Free Radical Research,* 37: 573-584.

Shahbazi Y (2017) The properties of chitosan and gelatine fluids incorporated with ethanolic red grape seed extract and *Ziziphora clinopodioides* essential oil as biodegradable materials for active food packaging. *International Journal of Biological Macromolecules*, 99: 746-753.

Sharma G, Tyagi AK, Singh RP, Chan DC, Agarwal R (2004) Synergistic anti-cancer effects of grape seed extract and conventional cytotoxic agent doxorubicin against human breast carcinoma cells. *Breast Cancer Res. Treat*. 85: 1–12.

Shinagawa FB, Santana FC, Torres LRO, Mancini-Filho J (2015) Grape seed oil: a potential functional food? *Food Science and Technology (Campinas)*, 35: 399-406.

Sineiro J, Dominguez H, Núñez MJ (1995) Pepitas de uva como fuente de aceite y proteína. Aliment. *Equipos Tecnol*. 14 : 49-56.

Stankovic M, Tesevic V, Vajs V, Todorovic N, Milosavljevic S, Godevac D (2008) Antioxidant properties of grape seed extract on human lymphocyte oxidative defence. *Planta Medica*, 74: 730-735.

Stoner GD, Mukhtar H (1995) Polyphenols as cancer chemopreventive agents, *J. Cell. Biochem*. 22: 169-180.

Tangolar SG, Özoğul Y, Tangolar S, Torun A (2009) Evaluation of fatty acid profiles and mineral content of grape seed oil of some grape genotypes. *International Journal of Food Sciences and Nutrition*, 60: 32-39.

Teixeira A, Baenas N, Dominguez-Perles R, Barros A, Rosa E, Moreno DA, Garcia-Viguera C (2014) Natural bioactive compounds from winery by-products as health promoters: a review. *International Journal of Molecular Sciences*, 15: 15638-15678.

Terra X, Valls J, Vitrac X, Mérrillon JM, Arola L, Ardèvol A., Bladé C, Fernandez-Larrea J, Pujadas G, Salvadó J, Blay M (2007) Grape-seed procyanidins act as anti-inflammatory agents in endotoxin-stimulated RAW 264.7 macrophages by inhibiting NF-κB signaling pathway. *Journal of Agricultural and Food Chemistry*, 55: 4357-4365.

Tociu M, Todasca M-C, Stanescu MD, Artem V, Ionescu V (2017) Climate impact on fatty acid content of grape seed oil. *UPB Scientific Bulletin Series B*, 79: 3-10.

Vijaimohan K, Jainu M, Sabitha K E, Subramaniyam S, Anandhan C, Shyamala Devi CS (2006) Beneficial effects of alpha linolenic acid rich flaxseed oil on growth performance and hepatic cholesterol metabolism in high fat diet fed rats. *Life Sciences*. 79(5): 448-454.

Vivancos M, Moreno JJ (2008) Effect of resveratrol, tyrosol and beta-sitosterol on oxidised low-density lipoprotein-stimulated oxidative stress, arachidonic acid release and prostaglandin E2 synthesis by RAW 264.7 macrophages. *Br J Nutr*. 99(6):1199–1207.

Wang J, Santa-Maria I, Ho L, Ksiezak-Reding H, Ono K, Teplow DB, Pasinetti GM (2010b) Inhibition of tau aggregation by grape derived polyphenols in a mouse model of Alzheimer's disease. *Journal of Alzheimer's Disease*, 22: 653-661.

Wang X, Tong H, Chen F, Gangemi JD (2010) Chemical characterization and antioxidant evaluation of muscadine grape pomace extract. *Food Chemistry*, 123: 1156-1162.

Wang YH, Yang XL, Wang L, Cui MX, Cai YQ, Li XL., Wu YJ (2010a) Effects of proanthocyanidins from grape seed on treatment of recurrent ulcerative colitis in rats. *Canadian Journal of Physiology and Pharmacology*, 88: 888-898.

Wattenberg LW (1996) Inhibition of tumorigenesis in animals. In: B. W. Stewart, D. McGregor, and P. Kleihues (eds.), *Principles of Chemo prevention*, pp. 151–159. Lyon, France: IARC.

Wen X, Zhu M, Hu R, Zhao J, Chen Z, Li J, Ni Y (2016) characterisation of seed oils from different grape cultivars grown in China. *Journal of Food Science and Technology*, 53: 3129-3136.

Yalcin H, Kavuncuoglu H, Ekici L, Sagdic O (2017) Determination of fatty acid composition, volatile components, physico-chemical and bioactive properties of grape (*Vitis vinifera*) seed and seed oil. *Journal of Food Processing and Preservation*, 41: e12854.

Yamaguchi F, Yoshimura Y, Nakazawa H, Ariga T (1999) Free radical scavenging activity of grape seed extract and antioxidants by electron spin resonance spectrometry in an H_2O_2/NaOH/DMSO system. *Journal of Agricultural and Food Chemistry*, 47: 2544-2548.

Yang T, Li X, Zhu W, Chen C, Sun Z, Tan Z, Kang J (2014) Alteration of antioxidant enzymes and associated genes induced by grape seed extracts in the primary muscle cells of goats *in vitro*. *PLoS ONE* 9(9): e107670. doi:10.1371/journal.pone.0107670.

Yemis O, Bakkalbasi E, Artik N (2008) Antioxidative activities of grape (*Vitis vinifera*) seed extracts obtained from different varieties grown in Turkey. *International Journal of Food Science and Technology*, 43: 154-159.

Yen C-Y, Hou M-F, Yang Z-W, Tang J-Y, Li K-T, Huang H-W, Huang Y-H, Lee S-Y, Fu T-F, Hsieh C-Y, Chen B-H, Chang H-W (2015) Concentration effects of grape seed extracts in anti-oral cancer cells involving differential apoptosis, oxidative stress and DNA damage. *BMC Complementary and Alternative Medicine*, 15: 94, DOI 10.1186/s12906-015-0621-8.

Yerlikaya P, Gokoglu N (2010) Inhibition effects of green tea and grape seed extracts on lipid oxidation in bonito fillets during frozen storage. *International Journal of Food Science and Technology*, 45: 252-257.

Yu J, Ahmedna M (2013) Functional components of grape pomace: their composition, biological properties and potential applications. *International Journal of Food Science and Technology*, 48: 221-237.

In: Seed Oil ISBN: 978-1-53613-560-2
Editor: Nguyen Khanh Dieu Hong

Chapter 5

ARGAN OIL: EXTRACTION, CATEGORIES, CHEMICAL COMPOSITION AND HEALTH BENEFITS

Wissal Dhifi[1], Maria da Graça Costa Miguel[2] and Wissem Mnif[3,4,*]

[1]LR17ES03 Physiopathologie, Alimentation et Biomolécules (PAB), Institut Supérieur de Biotechnologie de Sidi Thabet Biotechpole Sidi Thabet, Sidi Thabet, 2020, Université de La Manouba, Tunisie

[2]Department of Chemistry and Pharmacy, Laboratory of Chemistry of Natural Products, Faculty of Sciences and Technology, University of Algarve, Gambelas, 8005-139 Faro, Portugal

[3] Faculty of Sciences and Arts in Balgarn PO BOX 60 Balgarn- Sabt Al Olaya 61985, Bisha University, Saudi Arabia

[*] Corresponding author: Dr. Wissem Mnif, LR11-ES31 Laboratory of Biotechnology and Valorisation of Bio-GeoRessources, Higher Institute of Biotechnology of Sidi Thabet, BiotechPole of Sidi Thabet, 2020, Universiy of Manouba, Tunisia. Tel: + (216) 98 94 73 71. E-mail: w_mnif@yahoo.fr.

[4]Univ. Manouba, ISBST, BVBGR-LR11ES31, Biotechpole Sidi Thabet, 2020, Ariana, Tunisia

ABSTRACT

The Argan tree (*Arganiaspinosa* (L.) Skeels; Sapotaceae) is a slow-growing tree exclusively endemic to the barren lands of southwest Morocco. The oil extracted from argan seed is almost exclusively produced in southwestern Morocco. It is reputed for its unique savor and its several pharmacological and cosmetic properties.

The oil extraction requires a tedious multistep process. The first step is a careful fruit drying. This oil extraction requires a prolonged hand-malaxing of an aqueous argan kernel dow. The extraction yield can reach 35% and more. The extraction has been improved by the use of electric screw-presses, which allows the discontinuation of the hand-malaxing step, resulting in as much as 60-percent extraction yield.

Virgin edible argan oil is a main component of the Amazigh diet. It is prepared from slightly and carefully roasted kernels and it is copper-colored with a slight hazelnut taste. Health benefits of argan oil are attributed to its composition of unsaponiable fraction mainly rich in tocopherols. Argan oil has hepatoprotective, antiproliferative anti-diabetic properties and also cancer preventive potential. It is used in beauty and cosmetology since it has wound healer, anti-aging, anti-sebum, anti-acne and moisturizing properties.

Keywords: argan oil, chemical composition, cardiovascular prevention, cancer prevention, andiabetic effect

1. INTRODUCTION

The argan tree [*Arganiaspinosa* (L.) Skeels; Sapotaceae] is an 80-million-year-old relic tree species. The argan forest covers about 8,280 km2, mostly in the dry lowlands of the Souss valley and on the sunny mountain spurs of the Anti-Atlas. The argan tree grows very slowly. It takes fifteen years to mature. This tree can live for 150 years, and sometimes more than 200 years, and because of its deep root system, it can survive long periods of drought (Kenny et al., 2007; Morton et al., 1987). It constitutes the major source of Rural Amazigh families. Their life of any Amazigh family is strongly associated with the argan tree (Kenny et al., 2007; Benzyane et al., 1999). The oleaginous fruits of the argan tree furnish edible and marketable oil known as "argan oil", which provides up to 25% of the daily lipid diet for the local population and 9% of the annual oil production in Morocco (Benzyane et al., 1999).

Argan oil has rapidly emerged as the only product able to bring more wealth to the Berber population (Charrouf et al., 2008), the traditional argan forest dwellers, because of its unique dietary and physiological properties (Charrouf and Guillaume, 1999; Charrouf and Guillaume, 2008). Thus, prospects for better economic return have encouraged dwellers to modernize argan oil production methods for the export market.

2. Argan Oil Extraction

The extraction of argan oil is complex and influences significantly its physicochemical composition as well as its nutritional value and sensorial properties (Hilali et al., 2005). At present, two methods are used to extract argan oil for nutritional purposes: the traditional method (hand pressed) and a semi-industrial method (mechanical cold pressed) (Marfil et al., 2008). For many years, argan oil has been prepared exclusively by Berber women by a traditional multistep process (Charrouf et al., 2002). Some families collect up to six tons per season, others just a few hundred kilograms. The collect of fallen ripe fruit is done between May and August. Then the fruit is sun-dried for a few days, and the dried peel is removed manually to give argan nuts. To produce 60 kilograms of argan nuts approximately 100 kilograms of dried-fruit and 15 hours are needed. Argan nuts are then crushed between two stones, and the white kernels are collected. 6.5 kilograms of kernels are collected from 60 kilograms of argan nuts. To extract edible argan oil, kernels have to be roasted for a few minutes. It is worthy to notice that overheating should be avoided since it has a negative impact on the aroma and the taste of the oil. The roasted kernels are subsequently crushed using a millstone, thus giving a brownish viscous liquid that is mixed with water. This dough is hand-malaxed for several minutes, and it slowly becomes solid and releases an emulsion from which the argan oil is finally decanted (Matthaus et al., 2010).

The extraction residue or "press-cake" is dark-brown to black and generally, the hand-made extraction technique is very slow. In fact, ten hours are necessary for the production of one liter of oil. The raw oil is filtered and filled into bottles. Salt is added for its preservation (Charrouf and Guillaume, 1999).The mechanical extraction produces edible oil from roasted kernels, and oil for cosmetics and food supplements from unroasted kernels. The oil produced by hand-press extraction is characterized by a poor shelf-life (Charrouf and Guillaume, 1999). In the mechanical technique, kernel roasting is achieved in a rotating oven using gas burners. The introduction of the mechanical technique by several women cooperatives and industrial units improved not only the oil yield but also its quality. Thanks to the mechanical technique, the extraction time was significantly reduced (Charrouf and Guillaume, 1999). Despite all these advantages, the full process still remains slow and requires huge quantities of kernels. This justifies the expensive cost of argan oil (Charrouf et al., 2008).The mechanical extraction of argan oil can be classified in two means as follows:

- *Press extraction:* The mechanical press has been recently introduced to extract argan oil. In this technique, mixing of the dough and water is unnecessary and the dough can be directly pressed. The oil yield is of about 43%. Only two hours are needed to get one liter of oil.
- *Solvent extraction*: This technique is used for industrial or laboratory purposes (Hatinguais et al., 1983). One or two cycles of extraction are required. According to Charrouf (1984), the extraction yield is of 50 to 55%. Despite this advantage, this type of extraction furnishes an oil with organoleptic defaults compared to the traditional or press extraction according to Charrouf and Guillaume (1999). Since the oil produced by solvent extraction is

reserved for cosmetic uses, additives like tocopherols and polyphenols are incorporated.

3. Argan Oil Categories

Argan oils available on the market can be classified into two categories: cosmetic or edible oils. Both are virgin oils (cold-press). It is worthy to mention that cosmetic grade argan oil is prepared from non-roasted kernels whereas edible one is extracted by pressing slightly roasted kernels. This step dramatically modifies the taste of the edible oil and is responsible for its unique hazelnut taste and flavor. Traditionally, edible argan oil is eaten on bread. It is exploited as the principle fat source used for food preparation in the Amazigh diet and (Charrouf and Guillaume, 2010). Edible argan oil is also the main ingredient in Amlou, a Moroccan culinary specialty.

Some years ago cosmetic argan oil (INCI name: *Argania Spinoza* kernel oil) was sometimes extracted using volatile and lipophilic organic solvents (mostly hexane).Currently, such method is abandoned. Since it is extracted from non-roasted kernels, cosmetic argan oil is gold colored whereas edible argan oil is copper colored. Moreover, cosmetic argan oil is a non-fragrant oil. Its chemical composition is slightly different from that of edible argan oil (Hilali et al., 2005). Chemical investigation of the volatiles of edible and cosmetic argan oils has evidenced composition differences (Charrouf et al., 2006).

4. Argan Oil Chemical Composition

Virgin argan oil of edible or beauty grade is mainly composed of acyl glycerides (99%). This saponifiable fraction is mainly composed of triglycerides (TG) according to Charrouf and Guillaume (1999). The remaining fraction consists of the unsaponifiable matter, accounting for 1%

of the whole oil. The unsaponifiable fraction is composed of carotenes, tocopherols, triterpene alcohols, sterols, and xanthophylls (Chrarouf and Guillaume, 1999). The nutritional benefits of edible argan oil are due to its chemical composition. This oil is composed of upto 80%of unsaturated FA (18%) and of saturated FA (14%) as indicated in table 1. The major Fatty acids (FA) of argan oil are oleic C18: 1 and linoleic acid C18: 2 whose respective amounts are of 43-49% and 29-36% (Rahmani, 2005). Oleic acid is a monounsaturated FA of the omega-9 family, while linoleic acid is a polyunsaturated fatty acid belonging to the omega-6 family. Palmitic and stearic acids are saturated fatty acids found at concentrations of 11-15 percent and 4-7 percent, respectively (Rahmani, 2005).

Table 1. Chemical composition of argan oil (Guillaume and Charrouf, 2013)

Palmitic acid (C16 :0)	11.5-15%
Stearic acid (C18 :0)	4.3-7.2%
Oleic acid (C18:1 n-9)	43-49.1%
Linoleic acid (C18:2 n-6)	29.3-36%
Linolenic acid (C18 :3 n-3)	<0.3%
Total tocopherols	600-900 mg/kg
α-Tocopherol	2.4-6.5% of total
β-Tocopherol	0.1-0.3% of total
γ-Tocopherol	81-92% of total
δ-Tocopherol	6.2-12.8% of total
Total sterols	≤220mg/100g
Schottenol	44-49% of total
Spinasterol	34-44% of total
Δ7-avenasterol	4-7% of total

Argan oil is particularly rich in tocopherols, which are reputed as powerful antioxidants. Tocopherol content in argan oil can be up to 900 mg/ kg and is never below 600 mg/kg. Argan oil low content in linolenic acid and high content in tocopherol are likely to be responsible for its good stability (Guillaume and Charrouf, 2013). Argan oil phospholipids may participate in its preservation (Gharby et al., 2012). The amount of vitamin-E-active compounds in mechanically extracted argan oil generally varies from 400 to 775 mg/kg (Hilali et al., 2005) and is mainly composed of γ-tocopherol (Charrouf& Guillaume, 2007). According to Matthäus et al., (2010), argan oils contains approximately the same concentration of vitamin-E-active compounds after 20 weeks of storage. Furthermore, argan oil includes phenols such as vanillic acid, syringic acid, ferulic acid, tyrosol, catechol, resorcinol, (-)-epicatechin and (+)-catechin (Charrouf and Guillaume, 2007; Marfil et al., 2018).

Edible argan oil is also a rich source of Coenzyme Q10 and melatonin, two antioxidant molecules, but it does not seem to contain Coenzyme Q9. Only virgin soybean oil shows higher CoQ10 and melatonin levels than virgin argan oil (Venegas et al., 2011). Argan oil contains schottenol and spin sterol which are two sterols reputed for their anticancer properties (Arisawa et al., 1985; Villaseñor and Domingo, 2000). It also contains Campesterol at a low concentration close to 0.3% (Hilali et al., 2005).

5. Health Benefits of Argan Oil

Argan oil has several uses in a multiplicity of sectors (figure 1). Since argan oil is processed using a cold press, it retains a much larger amount of its nutritive components than oils pressed using a heated process. Thus, the particular chemical composition of argan oil confers to its significant health benefits. The high percentage of unsaturated FA and the important amount of tocopherols of argan oil are behind some of its pharmacological properties (Charrouf and Guillaume, 2008).

5.1. Cardiovascular Prevention

Hypolipidemic and hypocholesterolemic effects of argan oil have been demonstrated in rats. Blood lipoproteins were significantly due to the balanced composition of argan oil FA (Berrougui et al., 2003). Furthermore, argan oil is a source of powerful antioxidants which prevent cardiovascular diseases by inhibiting LDL-oxidation and enhancing reverse cholesterol transport (Berrougui et al., 2006). A daily intake of 25g of argan oil during 3 weeks resulted in a significant increase in high-density lipoprotein cholesterol (HDL) and apolipoprotein A-I as well as a decrease in triglycerides (Derouiche et al., 2005). This is in concordance with results of Drissi et al., (2004) who reported that argan oil consumers have lower levels of plasma LDL and cholesterol compared with the non-consumers. In addition, the triglycerides content of argan oil may have too cholesterol-lowering effects (Derouiche et al., 2005).

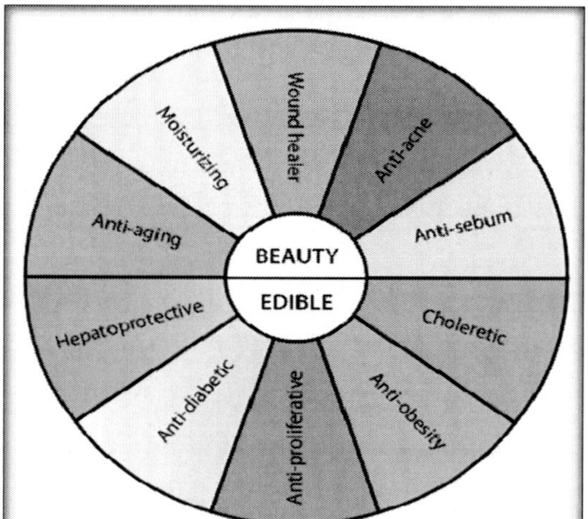

Figure 1. Therapeutic and cosmetic uses of argan oil (Guillaume and Charrouf, 2011).

The argan oil contains linoleic acid at a small amount. This FA produces prostaglandins, which play key role in immune system and circulation functions (Perdomo et al., 2011). Consumption of linoleic acid yields in an increased production of prostaglandins, which are beneficial for treatment of rheumatoid arthritis and cardio vascular problems (Semerano et al., 2011).

5.2. Cancer Prevention

Due to the similarity in the composition between olive and argan oils, an anti-proliferative effect has been claimed for argan oil (Khallouki et al., 2003). Argan oil is particularly rich in γ-tocopherol which is considered as a potent cancer chemo-preventive agent, more active than α-tocopherol (Gao et al., 2002; Huang et al., 2003).

Bennani (2009) reported that argan oil polyphenols exert a dose-dependent anti-proliferative action on two human epithelial cell lines PC3 and DPC1 cell lines. Furthermore, squalene in argan oil may act as protective against skin cancer (Newmark, 1997) and enhances excretion of xenobiotics in rats and mice (Kamimura et al., 1992).

5.3. Andiabetic Effect

According to Bnouham et al., (2008), argan oil reduced significantly the amount of absorbed glucose in perfused jejunum segment (2.5mL/Kg). Bellahcen et al., (2012) confirmed the antidiabetic effect of virgin argan oil. They reported a significant reduction of blood glucose and an important increase of hepatic glycogen level compared with the untreated rats diabetic group (Bellahcen et al., 2012). Further investigations should be done to explore the antidiabetic effect of argan oil in humans.

Conclusion

Argan constitutes a very precious bio-resource specific of the Maghreb and particularly of Morocco. It gives an oil with several health benefits and is valorized in cosmetic industry. Despite its multiple nutritional virtues, the consumption of argan oil remains limited. It should be encouraged. Further researches and investigations should be conducted to explore its properties in the human body and to understand its protective mechanisms against many diseases.

REFERENCES

Arisawa M., Kinghorn A.D., Cordell G.A., Phoebe C.H., Farnsworth N.R. (1985). Plant anticancer agents. XXXVI. Schottenol glucoside from *Baccharis cordifolia* and *Ipomopsis aggregata*. *Planta Medica*. 6: 544-545.

Bellahcen, S., Mekhfi, H., Ziyyat, A., Legssyer, A., Hakkou, A., Aziz, M., and Bnouham, M. (2012). Prevention of Chemically Induced Diabetes Mellitus in Experimental Animals byVirgin Argan Oil. *Phytother Res*. 26 (2):180-185.

Bennani, H. (2009). Impact of argan oil on prostate cancer Antiproliferative effect: study of polyphenols. *Rev Franco Lab*.416: 23-26.

Benzyane, M., Blerot, P., and Giot, P. (1999). *Le Grand Livre de la Forêt Marocaine* [The Great Book of the Moroccan Forest]; Mhirit, O., Blerot P., Eds.; Mardaga: Sprimont, Belgium, p. 280.

Berrougui, H., Cloutier, M., Isabelle, M., Khalil, A. (2006). Phenolic-extract from argan oil (*Arganiaspinosa* L.) inhibits human low-density lipoprotein (LDL) oxidation and enhances cholesterol efflux from human THP-1 macrophages. *Atherosclerosis*. 184 (2): 389–396.

Berrougui, H., Ettaib, A., Herrera Gonzalez, M.D., Alvarez de Sotomayor, M., Bennani-Kabchi, N. and Hmamouchi, M. (2003). Hypolipidemic and hypocholesterolemic effect of argan oil (*Arganiaspinosa* L.) in Meriones shawi rats. *J Ethnopharmacol*. 89 (1): 15–18.

Bnouham, M., Bellahcen, S., Benalla, W., Legssyer, A., Ziyyat, A., and Mekhfi, H. (2008). Antidiabetic activity assessment of Arganiaspinosa Oil. *J Complement Integr Med*. 5: 32.

Charrouf, Z., El Hamchi, H., Mallia, S., Licitra, G., and Guillaume, D. (2006). Influence of roasting and seed collection on argan oil odorant composition. *Nat Prod Commun*. 1: 399-404.

Charrouf, M. (1984). Contribution à l'étude chimique de l'huile *d'Argania spinosa* (L.) (sapotaceae). [Contribution to the chemical study of the oil of Argania spinosa (L.) (sapotaceae).] PhD Thesis, Perpignan, France.

Charrouf, Z. and Guillaume, D. (1999). Ethnoeconomical, ethnomedical, and phytochemical study of Argania spinosa (L.) Skeels. *J Ethnopharmacol*. 67: 7-14.

Charrouf, Z. and Guillaume, D. (2007). Phenols and polyphenols from *Argania spinosa. Amer J Food Tech.* 2: 679-683.

Charrouf, Z., Harhar, H., Gharby, S. and Guillaume, D. (2008). Enhancing the value of argan oil is the best mean to sustain the argan grove economy and biodiversity. *Oléagineux, Corps Gras, Lipides*, 15: 269–271.

Charrouf, Z. and Guillaume, D. (2008). Argan oil: Occurrence, composition and impact on human health. *Eur J Lipid Sci Technol.* 10 (7): 632–636.

Charrouf, Z. and Guillaume, D. (2010). Should the Amazigh diet (regular and moderate argan oil consumption) have a beneficial impact on human health? *Crit. Rev. Food Sci. Nutr*. 50 (5): 473-477.

Cherki, M., Berrougui, H., Drissi, A., Adlouni, A. and Khalil, A. (2006). Argan oil: which benefits on cardiovascular diseases? *Pharmacological Research*. 54 (1): 1–5.

Derouiche, A., Cherki, M., Drissi, A., Bamou, Y., El Messal, M., Idrissi-Oudghiri, A., et al. (2005). Nutritional intervention study with argan oil in man: effects on lipids and apolipoproteins. *Ann Nutr Metab. Karger Publishers*. 49 (3): 196–201.

Gao, R., Stone, W. L., Huang, T., Papas, A. M., and Qui, M. (2002). The uptake of tocopherols by RAW264.7 macrophages. *Nutrition Journal*. 1:2.

Gharby, S., Harhar, H., Guillaume, D., Haddad, A., Charrouf, Z. (2012). The origin of virgin argan oil's high oxidative stability unraveled. *Nat. Prod. Commun.* 7: 621-624.

Guillaume, D., and Charrouf, Z. (2011). Argan oil. *Alternative Medicine Review*, 16 (3): 275-279.

Guillaume, D., and Charrouf, Z. (2013). Argan oil for nutritional and skin care applications. *Agro Food Industry Hi Tech*. 24 (2): 28-30.

Hatinguais, P., Trebosc M. T. and Belle, R. (1983). Extrait lipidique du fruit de l'Arganier, procédé de préparation et application en cosmétologie. Fr. Patent FR2553 788-B1. p. 5.

Hilali, M., Charrouf Z., Soulhi, A. E. A., Hachimi, L., and Guillaume D. (2005). Influence of origin and extraction method on argan oil physico-chemical characteristics and composition. *Journal of Agricultural and Food Chemistry*. 53 (6): 2081–2087.

Huang, H. Y., Alberg, A. J., Norkus, E., Hoffman, S. C., Comstock, G. W., and Helzlsouer, K. J. (2003). Prospective study of antioxidant micronutrients in the blood and the risk of developing prostate cancer. *Am J Epidemiol*. 157: 335-344.

Kamimura, H., Koga, N., Oguri, K., and Yoshimura, H. (1992). Enhanced elimination of theophylline, phenobarbital and strychnine from the bodies of rats and mice by squalene tretment. *J pharmacobiodyn*. 15: 215-221.

Kenny, L., and De Zborowski, I. (2007). In *Atlas de l'arganier et de l'arganeraie* [Atlas of Argan and Argan Tree]; IAV Hassan II: Rabat, Morocco, 2007; p. 190.

Khallouki, F. (2003). *Ethnobotanical, Phytochemical and Pharmacological studies of 3 African medicinal plants containing potent antiradical principles*. PhD Dissertation, University of Metz, Metz, France.

Khallouki, F., Younos, C., Soulimani, R., Oster, T., Charrouf, Z., Spiegelhalder, B., et al. (2003). Consumption of argan oil (Morocco) with its unique profile of fatty acids, tocopherols, squalene, sterols and phenolic compounds should confer valuable cancer chemopreventive effects. *Eur J cancer Prev*. 12 (1): 67–75.

Marfil, R., Cabrera-Vique, C., Giménez, R., Bouzas, P.R., Martínez, O., Sánchez, J. A. (2008). Metal Content and physicochemical parameters used as quality criteria in virgin argan oil: Influence of the extraction method. *J Agric Food Chem*. 56: 7279- 7284.

Morton, J. F., and Voss, G. L. (1987). The Argan Tree (*Argania sideroxylon*, Sapotaceae), A Desert Source of Edible Oil. *Econ*. 41: 221-233.

Newmark, H. L. (1997). Squalene, olive oil, and cancer risk: a review and hypothesis. *Cancer Epidemiol Biomarkers Prevention*. 6: 1101-1103.

Perdomo, M., Santos, J. E., and Badinga, L. (2011). Trans-10, cis-12 conjugated linoleic acid and the PPAR-γ agonist rosiglitazone attenuate lipopolysaccharide-induced TNF-α production by bovine immune cells. *Dom Animal Endocrinol*. 41: 118-125.

Rahmani, M. (2005). The chemical composition of virgin argan oil. *Agricultures*. 14: 461-465.

Semerano, L., Clavel, G., Assier, E., Denys, A., and Boissier, M. C. (2011). Blood vessels, a potential therapeutic target in rheumatoid arthritis? *Joint Bone Spine*. 78: 118-123.

Venegas, C., Cabrera-Vique, C., García-Corzo, L., Escames, G., Acuña-Castroviejo, D., López, L. C. (2011). Determination of coenzyme Q10, coenzyme Q9, and melatonin contents in virgin argan oils: Comparison with other edible vegetable oils. *J. Agric. Food Chem*. 59: 12102–12108.

Villaseñor, I. M., and Domingo, P. (2000). Anticarcinogenicity potential of spinasterol isolated from squash flowers. *Teratogenesis, Carcinogenesis, and Mutagenesis*. 20: 99-105.

In: Seed Oil ISBN: 978-1-53613-560-2
Editor: Nguyen Khanh Dieu Hong

Chapter 6

RUBBER SEED OIL: PROPERTIES, USES AND BENEFITS

Nguyen Khanh Dieu Hong[1,*], Nguyen Dang Toan[1], Dinh Thi Ngo [1], Dao Sy Duc[2] and Ta Ngoc Don[1]

[1]Hanoi University of science and technology, Hanoi, Vietnam
[2]VNU University of Science, Hanoi, Vietnam

ABSTRACT

Rubber seed oil is considered as second-generation feedstock that could play a crucial role in many applications including biofuel, bio-lubricant, detergent, paints and coating, etc. This chapter will provide an overview from properties to applications of the rubber seed oil. Some of our research achievement relating to application of the rubber seed oil in biodiesel synthesis will be also described.

Keywords: rubber seed oil, biodiesel, application, second-generation

* Corresponding Author Email: dieuhongprof@gmail.com.

INTRODUCTION

Rubber seed oil (RSO), produced from the seeds of *Hevea brasiliensis*, through press and extraction processes, is a renewable and sustainable source which could be used in many applications including biodiesel synthesis because of its second generation, inedible and high productivity feedstock. Furthermore, it can be injected directly into an internal-combustion engine (Geo et al. 2008), or blended with diesel derived from fossil crude oil (Ramadhas et al. 2005). RSO can be also transferred into methyl esters, ethyl esters, in methanolysis process based on many trans-esterification procedures (Ikwuagwu et al. 2000; Melvin et al. 2011; Satyanarayana et al. 2010; Khan et al. 2010; Ramadhas et al. 2005), over different types of catalysts (Yang et al. 2011). In order to improve the fuel performance, RSO and its methyl esters can be inducted by hydrogen (Geo et al. 2009) or coir-pith producer gas (Ramadhas et al. 2008), or mixed with diethyl ether (Geo et al. 2010). The performance and emissions of RSO biodiesel have been tested (Ramadhas et al. 2005) and compared with other vegetable based biodiesels (Satyanarayana et al. 2011; Yusup et al. 2010) and found to be a suitable source for biodiesel production at large scale. Satyanarayana et al. (Satyanarayana et al. 2011) found that the RSO is not only a reliable choice for producing biodiesel fuel, but also one of the sources with the lowest CO_2 and NO_2 emission rates.

Other applications of the RSO can be considered including alkyd resins (Aigbodion et al. 2000; Aigbodion 2003; Ong et al. 2016), soap cakes, detergent and surfactant (Ohikhena et al. 2006; Aiwize et al. 2012; Osagie et al. 2014), lubricants (Kamalakar et al. 2013; Aravind et al. 2016), paints and coatings, vanish, surfactants and biodiesel (Ikwuagwu et al. 2000; Singh et al. 2017), etc.

The oil content of the rubber seeds can change from 50 to 60% and of kernel from 40 to 50% of oil. These oils can contain a high content of free fatty acids (FFAs) which may up to 17% wt (Atabani et al. 2013). The oil has high content of the unsaturated FFAs, for example linoleic (~39%), oleic (~25%), and linolenic (~16%) acids (Kumar and Sharma, 2011).

Over the world, the RSO plantations requires landscapes of 9,712,355.52 ha (Wu et al. 2010). Wu et al. also states that China and many other countries should focus on inedible biomass for biodiesel production in the near future; then they can positively choose the RSO as an alternative candidate for the traditional sources. Actually, there are some calculations for potential of the RSO based on the amounts of rubber seeds produced per hectare in many areas in Asia including Southeast Asia, Indian, Malaysia, Bangladesh and China for many years. Results show that China has a vast increase in the RSO productivity during 1999 to 2005 caused by the previous given reason (Ramadhas et al. 2005; Melvin et al. 2011; Ramadhas et al. 2005; Jamieson et al. 1930; Gandhi et al. 1990; Morshed et al. 2011; Jianbai et al. 2004-1; Jianbai et al. 2004-2; Zhao et al. 2008; Xiankun et al. 2009; Qianwen et al. 1999; Weiwei et al. 2005).

In Vietnam, according to the Vietnam Rubber Group, the RSO plant is mainly distributed in the South with area above 500,000 ha (up to ~ 1,000,000 ha considering to expanded plants growing in Laos and Cambodia) expected to produce 330,000 tons of oil per year for main applications in paint and lacquer industry (Hong et al. 2016; Dat et al. 2012). The RSO is considered as the second-generation feedstock with favorable chemical components for biodiesel production demonstrated by many publications (Eka et al. 2010; Lin et al. 2010; Ramadhas et al. 2005). Some studies consider an occurrence of a toxic compound (Linamarin) in its component avoiding the uses of the RSO in food processing (Dat et al. 2012; Ramadhas et al. 2005). As a consequence, the application of the RSO in biodiesel production was indicated as a sustainable way to develop the production of alternative fuels in Vietnam.

Properties of RSO

Fatty Acid Profile

The RSO belongs to semidrying oil group and has yellow or pale brown color. Its composition contains a large amount of unsaturated fatty acids having total molar ratio of about 4/1 to saturated ones – a very specific rates of the RSO. The most important fatty acids in the RSO consist of oleic acid (C18:1), linoleic acid (C18:2), linoleic acid (C18:3) belonging to the unsaturated group, and palmitic acid (C16:0), stearic acid (C18:0) belonging to the saturated one; in which the oleic and linoleic content takes higher than 80% by weight. Therefore, the RSO can be considered as a typical oleic-linoleic vegetable oil (Yong et al. 2006).

Actually, the RSO has been less applicable compared to many other edible oils such as soybean, sunflower… oils because of many reasons. One of the main reasons is that its composition contains many FFAs, so in many applications such as paint and coating, lubricant, biodiesel fuel, it is very important to reduce or remove these components (Carraretto et al. 2004). Other reason relates to some toxic compounds exist in the RSO, for example, some cyanides and porphobilinogens, which seriously destroy blood cells (Iyayi et al. 2008; Gabien et al. 1990). The RSO cannot be used in the food industry for human. Its composition extracted from some kind of the RSO can be brifted in Table 1.

The statistic exhibits that there is minor difference among the unsaturated and saturated fatty acid contents of different type of the RSOs, reflecting a stable rate in the RSO from many regions. However, the FFA contents can be very different with each kind of the RSO (Abdullah et al. 2009).

The fatty acid components mainly distribute in triglycerides (TAGs), which have been studied for their composition and structure in some researches. Table 2 describes many kinds of the TAGs existed in the Malaysian RSO.

Being well-suited with the previous given compositions, this component contains many unsaturated TAGs leading to some negative effects during storing time of the RSO. The RSO therefore possess quite low stability which need to be well reserved in appropriate conditions.

Table 1. Fatty acid composition of the RSO

Fatty acids, %wt	Malaysia RSO	Nigeria RSO
Myristic ($C_{14:0}$)	2.2	-
Palmitic ($C_{16:0}$)	8.56 ± 0.07	17.51
Stearic ($C_{18:0}$)	10.56 ± 0.02	4.82
Oleic ($C_{18:1}$)	22.95 ± 0.15	25.33
Linoleic ($C_{18:2}$)	37.28 ± 0.10	37.50
Linoleic ($C_{18:3}$)	19.22 ± 0.21	14.21
Saturated acids	19.12 ± 0.28	22.33
Unsaturated acids	79.45 ± 0.31	77.04
Free oleic acid	7.55 ± 0.02	21.40

Table 2. TAG composition in Malaysian RSO

TAGs	Number of carbon	*Content, % wt*
LnLnLn	36	2,3
LnLnL	38	7,7
LnLL	40	5,9
LLL	42	4,1
OLLn	42	5,9
PLLn	42	3,9
PLL	44	5,8
LnOP	44	1,7
LnOO	44	7,5
POL + SOL	46	3,3
POO	48	1,9
PPL	46	6,4
POP	48	4,4
POS	50	1,0
PPP	48	3,9

Ln: linolenic acid ($C_{18:3}$); L: linoleic acid ($C_{18:2}$); O: oleic acid ($C_{18:1}$); P: palmitic acid ($C_{16:0}$); S: stearic acid ($C_{18:0}$).

Acid Value

The acid value of the RSO, as mentioned above, is high and variable in different kinds of the oils (Asuquo et al. 2010; Abdullah et al. 2009). Acid value is calculated based on amount of potassium hydroxide (mg) needed to neutralize the FFAs (in one gram of the oil). The lower the acid value of an oil, the fewer FFAs it contains which makes it less exposed to the phenomenon of rancidification (Asuquo et al. 2010). Acid value varies according to the extraction method with high acidity by Soxhlet method because of the onset of oxidation, but most of the case relates to the existence of lipase enzyme in the composition of the RSOs which can gradually hydrolyze the oil (Asuquo et al. 2010). Acid value, therefore, can be used to test the level of oxidative effects of the oil by enzymatic or chemical impacts.

Saponification Value

Saponification value can be determined by measurement of the mass of potassium hydroxide (in mg) needed to neutralize all the FFAs and saponify the esters contained in 1 g of the lipid (Asuquo et al. 2010). Asuquo et al. points that the saponification value of the RSO is about 193.61, compared to that of common oils such as soybean (189 – 195), peanut (187 – 196) and cotton seed (189 – 198). Other study state that the saponification value of the RSO is about 182.12 ± 0.27 mg/g being similar to the other typical seed oil such as sunflower or corn (O’Brien 2004) and lower than the other ones such as coconut, palm kernel seed, or higher than castor (Basbes et al. 2004), and perah (Yong et al. 2006; Gunstone et al. 1994).

Unsaponifiable Matter

The unsaponifiable matter is also important to determine the whole quantity of compounds which exist in the oil as well as the quality of oil. The value of unsaponifiable matter of RSO is 1.83 ± 0.01 % (Table 1). This value is in agreement with the value reported in by (Ghandhi et al. 1990).

Toxicity

Toxicity of the RSO mainly comes from the cyanides characterized by occurrence of -CN groups in the oil composition (Toda et al. 2005; Roman et al. 2003; Ghana Statistical Service 2011). One of the most available compound owning this kind of the group is linamarine (Figure 1):

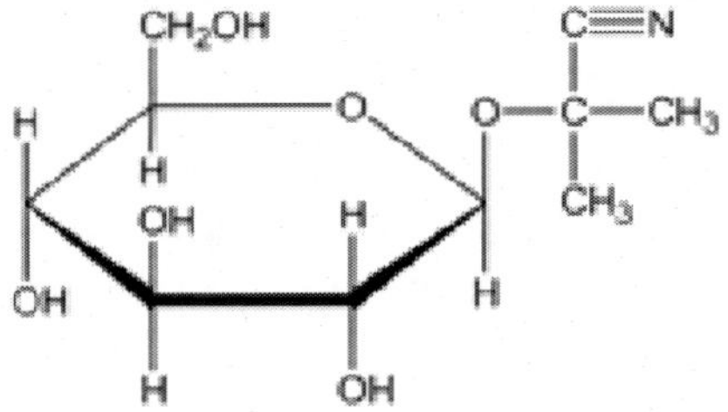

Figure 1. Structure of linamarine.

Linamarine, possessing high toxicity, cancinogernic, combining with the high content of the FFAs, makes the RSO as a typical inedible oil. The RSO cannot be used in food technology, but can be very useful in other mentioned industrial applications.

Other Properties

Refractive index (RI) of the RSO can reach 1.4-1.6, according to (Kovo et al. 2007). The value belongs to a common range of the refractive index assigned for many vegetable oils such as castor seed (1.47), sterculia setegera (1.46), blighia sapida (1.45) and shear butter (1.60) (Asuquo et al. 2010; Kyari et al. 2008). RI can be considered as an indication of the level of saturation in the vegetable oils.

The pH value of the RSO is approximately of 5.8-6.0 proving its acidity because of its high content of the FFAs. This pH value is considerable higher than this of other vegetable edible oils such as soybean, rapeseed, etc. (Aremu et al. 2008). However, the acidity of the oil can be advantageous in utilization of the oil in soap making when the neutralization of the FFAs is much more convenient than of the TAGs. The viscosity of the RSO, because of the FFAs occurrence, is slightly lower than those of other oils, e.g., castor oil, shear butter oil and crambe oil (Asuquo et al. 2010).

The specific gravity of RSO was found to be 0.92 indicating that the oil is less dense than water. Also, the value seems to indicate that no heavy element is present in the oil (Aigbodion et al. 2005). The specific gravity obtained for RSO in this study is similar to those of other oils e.g., shea butter oil (0.92) and castor seed oil (0.96) (Asuquo et al. 2008). High specific gravity is caused by the presence of hydroxyl groups as found in castor oil. Aigbodion and Bakare (Aigbodion et al. 2005) reported a specific gravity of 0.916 for RSO obtained from the rubber research institute of Nigeria.

Peroxide value of 14.4 was obtained for RSO in one study (Asuquo 2012). Peroxide value is an indication of deterioration of oils. Oils with higher peroxide values are more unsaturated than those with lower peroxide values. More unsaturated oils are known to absorb more oxygen and develop higher peroxide values, and oils with higher peroxide values are prone to rancidity (Asuquo et al. 2008).

Iodine value is also an important property of the RSO because it measures the degree of unsaturation in the oil. The iodine value also indicates whether or not the oil can be stable in the oxidation environment (air). It determines the stability of oils to oxidation, and allows the overall unsaturation of the fat to be determined qualitatively (Asuquo 2010). The iodine value of the RSO can range from 130 to 140 proving that the oil is not a stable candidate compared to the others (Asuquo et al. 2008; Abdullah et al. 2009).

The ester value, different from the saponification value, represents the percentage of esters in the RSO, namely, the ester value is a subtract of the saponification value to the acid value. With the RSO, the ester value can range from 187-192, being higher than those shear butter oil (183), and castor oil (174) (Asuquo 2010).

APPLICATIONS OF RSO

Rubber seed is obtained in high yield as a by-product of *Hevea* cultivated primarily for its latex. Its traditional use is as planting material. However, research has shown it to be a rich source of oil that is comparable in quality to dry oils commonly used in surface coatings (Aremu et al. 2008; Aigbodion et al. 2005); Asuquo et al. 2008; Asuquo et al. 2012). RSO is therefore considered as an attractive candidate for development to supplement current supply of vegetable oils in the country. There are many applications could be required the RSO as a beginning, intermediate or additive material, including alkyd resin, detergent, lubricant, biodiesel, etc.

Alkyd Resins

In a study, Aigbodion et al. (Aigbodion et al. 2000) apply the RSO in the manufacture of alkyd resins (both solvent- and water-borne) which are evaluated as binders in air-drying surface coatings. Also, RSO was modified by heating and evaluated as binders in surface coatings. Water-borne RSO alkyds seem promising in production of low volatile organic component (VOC), non-polluting and environmentally friendly coatings. These represent new areas of application of RSO, and development of water-borne RSO alkyds is consistent with the global trend aimed at reduction of VOC of coatings. For the feedstock using in the study, its acid value of 53 is very high corresponding to about 26.5% wt of FFAs in the oil. Results indicate that the synthesized alkyd samples are well resistant to water and alkali.

Later study of Aigbodion et al. (Aigbodion 2003) develops the process in the other way: The RSO as a renewable resource was used in the production of alkyd emulsion instead of neat resin. The RSO is initially treated with different amounts of maleic anhydride. The maleinized RSO is then used to generate water-soluble alkyd sample. The sample and their original alkyd are evaluated for their physico-chemical properties and compared to the pure RSO. Acid, saponification and iodine values are affected by maleinization. The product contains lower volatile organic compound (VOC) (between 1 and 1.5%) compared to its corresponding alkyd resin (about 10%). The product also exhibited excellent resistance to acid, brine and water, and fair resistance to alkali.

Ong et al. (Ong et al. 2016) discover bioresin prepared from RSO via alcoholysis–polyesterification process over homogeneous base catalyst tailored by CuO nanoparticles. The polyesterification process was controlled by varying the acid values as a function of time at different CuO nanoparticle concentrations. The formation of the alkyd resin is confirmed as well as the addition of CuO nanoparticles into the process greatly improve the reaction for synthesizing the bioresin from vegetable oil while reducing the reaction time. Besides, the antimicrobial properties in the resin are also considerable strengthen.

Detergents

Detergent means soap produced from the RSO. There are many works trying to do and to improve this process. Ohikhena (Ohikhena et al. 2006) use the RSO having high acid value, inedible and average saponification value in soap manufacture. On the other site, a substitution is applied by using palm kernel oil in the production of soaps (bar soap and detergent soap). Tests for the foam capacity and stability of these soaps exhibited good visual foam stabilities and capacities of both types from the two feedstocks. Therefore, soap from the RSO can be suitable for washing and cleaning.

Aiwize et al. (Aiwize et al. 2012) investigate for optimum blend ratio of RSO to palm kernel oil (PKO) for making soap, and find out the RSO:PKO of 20:80 being constituent elements used for the production of the soap.

Osagie et al. (Osagie et al. 2014) also produce soap using RSO and alkali derived from cassava peels ash extract. The soap is analysed to determine it chemical composition and efficacy. The result obtained in this research has shown that soap with similar characteristic and washing efficiency can be produced using locally source materials from agricultural waste and non-edible oil. The soap, if well prepared, can be used as a cheap source for industrial cleaning agent synthesis.

Lubricants

Kamalakar et al. (Kamalakar et al. 2013) use RSO containing palmitic 9.3%; stearic 8.4%; oleic 25.4%; linoleic 41.1% and linolenic 15.3% acids, for preparation of lubricant base stocks. The oil is hydrolyzed in the first step to produce obtain fatty acids followed by reacting with 2-ethyl-1-hexanol (2-EtH) and neopentyl glycol (NPG), trimethylolpropane (TMP), pentaerythritol (PE) at 135–140°C in the presence of p- toluene sulfonic acid (p-TSA) as catalyst in xylene medium. The branched and polyol esters were obtained in the range of 91–96.5% yields. The esters are considered as lubricant stock base after passing many tests including kinematic viscosity, viscosity index, copper corrosion, oxidative stability (RBOT), weld load, wear, pour and flash points. Among the base stocks prepared, polyol esters were found to possess good viscosity indices (205–222) compared to branched esters (187). Good weld load behavior was observed in the case of PE (170 kg) and TMP (160 kg) esters compared to NPG (130 kg) and 2-ethyl-1-hexanol (120 kg) esters. All the esters exhibited good copper corrosion values of 1a. The study revealed that all the esters can be well exploited for a number of hydraulic fluid formulations.

Aravind et al. (Aravind et al. 2016) also synthesize biolubricant from the rich free fatty acid RSO harvested from Kerala, India. Many properties of the feedstock and product are tested including pour point, cloud point, flash point, acid value, saponification value, viscosity, viscosity index etc. The results reveal that the presence of densed double bonds in the oil yielding in suitable epoxidation which is favourable for the lubricant properties.

Biodiesel

Ikwuagwu et al. (Ikwuagwu et al. 2000) synthesize biodiesel from the RSO after being bleached, through transesterification with 6-molar excess of methanol using sodium hydroxide as a catalyst. Methyl ester yield and fuel properties of the oil and product are determined and compared to that of commercial diesel fuel. The analysis of the properties in comparison to commercial diesel fuel shows that the transmethylation strongly improves the fuel properties of the oil. The viscosity substantially reduces from 37.85 to 6.29 cSt. Calculated cetane index increases from 34.00 to 44.81 and other properties are also found to be improved. The results supports the choice of monoesters, in place of straight RSO, as having better potential for use as alternative fuel.

Singh et al. (Singh et al. 2017) studies process for refining RSO as a feedstock in biodiesel production. The refining has purpose in removal of impurities such as peroxides and high oxidative components that not only affect the oil stability, colour and shelf-life but promote insoluble gums formation with time that could cause deposition in the combustion engines. Degumming and bleaching are the two applied processes. The analysis of variance shows that bleaching earth dosage was the most influencing factor followed by reaction time and phosphoric acid dosage. The results show a reduction in the peroxide value of the oil. The optimum reaction conditions gives the reduction of the peroxide value up to 0.1 meq/g. This was achieved at 40 wt% of bleaching earth dosage, at a reaction time of 20 min with 1 wt% of phosphoric acid usage.

Morshed et al. (Morshed et al. 2011) report that in their paper, RSO is investigated as a potential source for biodiesel production in Bangladesh. Biodiesel is prepared using a three-step method comprises with saponification of oil, acidification of the soap and esterification of FFAs. Overall yield of FFA from RSO is around 86%. The final step is esterification that produces fatty acid methyl ester (FAME). The effect of methanol to oil ratio and catalyst content has been investigated for esterification reaction. The results indicate that at optimum conditions, 98% conversion of the FFA to FAME is obtained. Biodiesel properties are determined proving a significant reduction of viscosity and acid value. Other properties, such as specific gravity, viscosity, flash point, cloud point, pour point and calorific value are comparable with the petrodiesel.

Roschat et al. (Roschat et al. 2017) present biodiesel production from RSO in Thailand. 24 wt% of oil is successfully extracted from the rubber seed powder using hexane (0.5 v/wt of solvent/seed ratio). This high FFAs oil (>3 wt%) was successfully transesterified by various heterogeneous catalysts such as CaO-based waste coral fragment, sodium metasilicate and CaO-based eggshell to biodiesel in high yield and high % FAME. The RSO biodiesel can be collected without any treatment and cleaning process shows high quality fuel properties that satisfy all EN 14214 and high-speed diesel standards.

Other studies also strongly confirm that biodiesel production from RSO is completely potential under suitable conditions and catalysts. These studies can be counted as Onoji et al. 2016; Ahmad et al. 2014; Qin Ng et al. 2013; and Zhu et al. 2014.

OUR RESULTS IN BIODIESEL SECTOR

Cellulose Based Catalyst for Converting the RSO to Biodiesel

The esterification of higher fatty acids by liquid acid catalysts such as sulfuric acid (H_2SO_4) was a process commonly used for biodiesel production, but it involved high consumption of energy, and separation of the catalysts from the homogeneous reaction mixtures was costly and chemically wasteful. Recyclable solid acids, for example, the Nafion (Okuhara et al. 2002; Smith et al. 2003), were better candidates, although they are also expensive and their relatively low activity compared to that of liquid acids. There are some other solid acids described as they possessed great activity on both esterification and trans-esterification such as SO_6^{2-}/ZrO_2, acid supported mesoporous materials (Camila et al. 2008; Yan et al. 2010; Alexandre et al. 2010; Juan et al. 2009). However, these catalysts required extreme conditions for well converting feedstock to methyl esters, even when they were categorized as super acids.

Carbon-based or biomass-based catalysts were a relatively novel, advanced and important class of the solid catalysts. Discovery of the sugar catalyst by Toda et al. in 2005 had attracted considerable interest because it could be prepared from renewable sources such as sugars, starch and cellulose, using low energy in the pyrolysis step (carbonization temperature ~400°C) for precursor preparations, and ease of functionalization of the carbon-based surface by sulfonating in sulfuric acid to produce the acid catalysts. Furthermore, activity and selectivity of the sugar catalyst was comparable with sulfuric acid for both the esterification and trans-esterification reactions (Toda et al. 2005).

According to Toda et al. a glucose based solid acid was prepared through two-step process including partial carbonization of D-glucose followed by sulfonation of the carbonized powder. The catalyst exhibited considerable activity on methanolysis because of the introduction of $-SO_3H$ groups on its surface. However, there were a few information relating to the structure of the catalyst published in that paper, and a conclusion about potential of widening the materials such as starch and cellulose for catalyst preparation was not demonstrated. In the field of our works, we also realized that the catalysts prepared from sugar, starch or cellulose or even natural biomass by the given two-step process also possessed high density of sulfonic acid ($-SO_3H$) groups generating the superacid sites and exhibited great activity in methanolysis of a wide range of feedstock. The catalyst consisted of flexible polycyclic carbon nanosheets with acid groups such as $-SO_3H$, -COOH, and phenolic hydroxyl (-OH) in a three-dimensional network (Toda et al. 2005).

For the feedstock aspect, the RSO was considered as the second-generation feedstock with favorable chemical components for biodiesel production demonstrated by a lot of publications. The composition of the RSO included a large amount of FFAs contributed by the oil sources and the existence of lipase catalyzed hydrolysis of the TAGs, so various base catalysts could not be applied for the conversion because of saponification during the synthesis. As mentioned above the best way in this case was to develop a new solid acid catalyst with high activity and selectivity (superacid). Hence the carbon-based catalysts were considered as potential candidates to overcome this challenge.

Our works belonged to a large group studying preparation, characterization and application of carbon-based catalysts derived from many sources such as sugars, starch, cellulose, waste biomass, etc. in the biodiesel synthesis from different rich FFA vegetable oils including RSO, microalgae oil and deodorizer distillate. This report covered some new approaches including preparation of a carbon-based catalyst derived from cellulose, so called cellulose based catalyst, demonstration of the $-SO_3H$ attached on the polycyclic aromatic system and application of the as-synthesized catalyst for converting the Vietnam RSO to biodiesel.

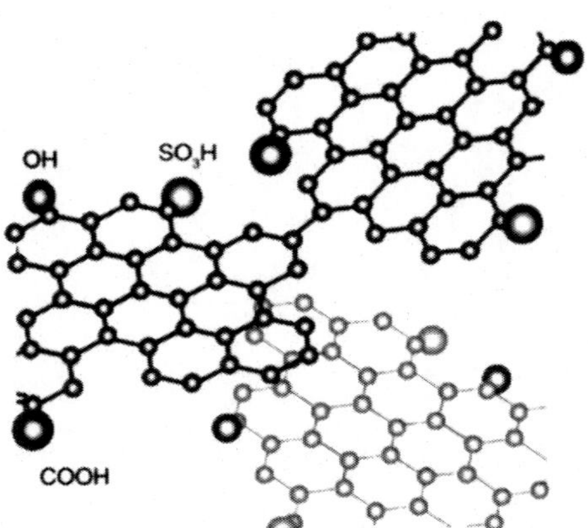

Figure 2. Structure of carbon based catalyst according to Toda.

Cellulose based catalyst was prepared through a two-step procedure including partial cellulose carbonization at 400°C for 2 hours to obtain "black powder," and sulfonation of the black powder using concentrated sulfuric acid at 230°C for 16 hours to synthesize the catalyst. The as-synthesized catalyst possessed super acid sites assigned for – SO_3H groups located on polycyclic aromatic fragments enhancing its activity on methanolysis of a wide range of vegetable oils and animal fats. In this study, the activity of the catalyst was demonstrated on the Vietnamese RSO containing a large amount of the FFAs in its chemical composition for synthesizing the fatty acid methyl esters (FAMEs) known as biodiesel. The methanolysis were established at 130°C in an autoclave reactor, and the reaction reached a yield of 95.8% after 4 hours. Some properties of the RSO were determined by various standard methods and described in Table 3.

Table 3. Some RSO specifications

Properties	Methods	Values
Density (25°C)	D 1298	0.925
Kinetic viscosity at 40°C, cSt	D 445	60
Pouring point, °C	D 97	-20
Saponification value, mg KOH/g	D 464	198
Acid number, mgKOH/g	D 664	67
Iodine number, g I_2/100g	EN 1411	142.8
Flash point, °C	D 93	220.2
Water content, mg/kg	D 95	253
Residue content, mg/kg	EN 12622	245
Carbon residue content, mg/kg	D 189	19
High heating value, MJ/Kg	D 2015	35.3
Refractive index	E 2583	1.4712
Color	-	Transparent, heavy brown
Odor	-	Specific

The acid number of the RSO was very high (67) responding for about 33.5% of the FFAs, do the base catalysts was unable to use in the methanolysis because of the saponification. The methanolysis on the cellulose-based catalyst completely avoided the saponification, so this was a very suitable way to do with various kinds of feedstock. The highest yield of biodiesel was 95.8% after 4 hours of reaction demonstrating a great activity of the catalyst. The refined biodiesel obtained from the methanolysis was analyzed by GC-MS method to determine the fatty acid methyl ester (FAMEs) composition and described in Figure 3 and Table 4. The FAMEs content reached 100.00% demonstrating a very high purity of the refined biodiesel.

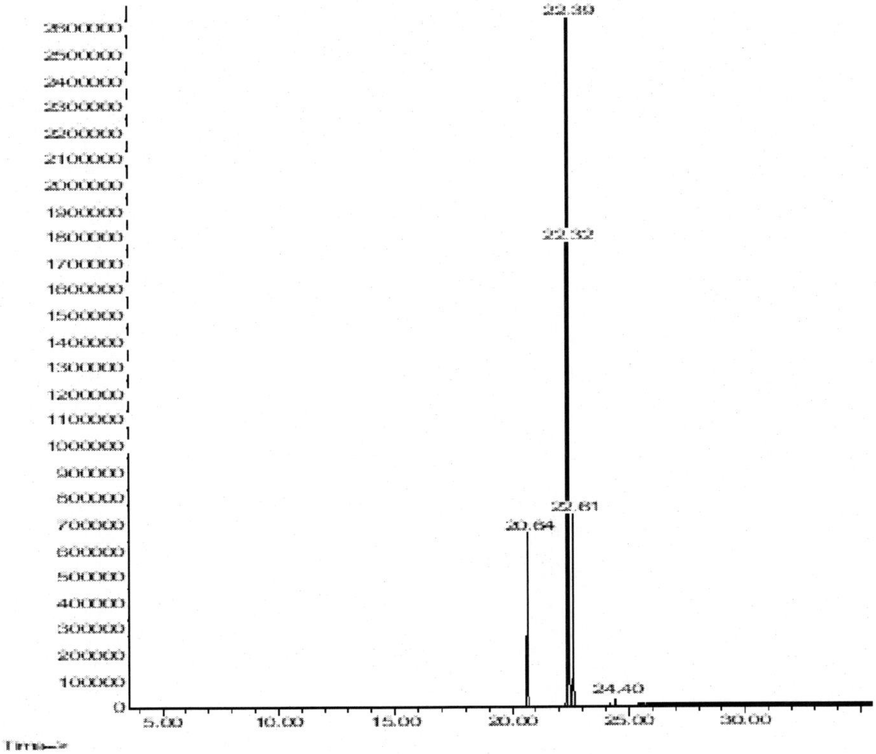

Figure 3. GC diagram of the refined biodiesel.

Table 4. Fatty acid composition in refined biodiesel derived from GC-MS results

No.	Acid names	Components	Formulas	Contents, %
1	Hexadecanoic	C16:0	$C_{16}H_{32}O_2$	10.69
2	9,12-Octadecadienoic	C18:2	$C_{18}H_{32}O_2$	28.90
3	13-Octadecenoic	C18:1	$C_{18}H_{34}O_2$	47.79
4	Octadecanoic	C18:0	$C_{18}H_{36}O_2$	12.12
5	Eicosanoic	C20:0	$C_{20}H_{40}O_2$	0.50
Sum				100.00

REFERENCES

Abdullah B. M., Salimon O. 2009. "Physicochemical characteristics of Malaysian rubber (Hevere brasiliensis) seed oil." *Eur. J. Sci. Rej* 31:431-445.

Aigbodion A. I., Bakare I. O. 2005. "Rubber seed oil quality assessment and authentification." *J. Am. Oil Chem. Soc* 82:465-469.

Aigbodion A. I., Okieimen F. E., Obazee E. O., Bakare I. O. 2003. "Utilisation of maleinized rubber seed oil and its alkyd resin as binders in water-borne coatings." *Progress in Organic Coatings* 46:28–31.

Aigbodion A. I., Pillai C. K. S. 2000. "Preparation, analysis and applications of rubber seed oil and its derivatives in surface coatings." *Progress in Organic Coatings* 38:187–192.

Aiwize E. A., Achebo J. I. 2012. "Liquid soap production with blends of rubber seed oil (RSO) and palm kernel oil (PKO) with locally sourced caustic potash (KOH)." *Nigerian Journal of Technology (NIJOTECH)* 31(1):63-67.

Alexandre D., Gadi R. 2010. *"Sulfated zirconia catalyst." its production by melting the precursors and its use for esterification of fatty acids with alcohols* WO 2010/010118 A1.

Amith Aravind, K. Prabhakaran Nair, M. L. Joy. 2016. "Physio-Chemical Characterization of Rubber Seed Oil (Hevea brasiliensis)-A

Biodegradable Lubricant Substitute." *Technology Letters ISSN: 2348-8131* 3(2):20-24.

Aremu, M. O., Olaofe, O., Atolaiye, B. O., Amos, V. A. 2008. "The physicochemical properties and fatty acid composition of sponge luffa (Luffa cylindrica) kernel oils." In: *Proceedings of the Chemical Society of Nigeria.* Petroleum Training Institute, Effurum-Warri, Delta State, Nigeria.

Asuquo J. E. 2008. *"Studies on the Adsorption of Some Selected Metallic Soaps onto Hematite."* Ph.D. Dissertation, University of Port Harcourt, Nigeria.

Asuquo J. E., Anusiem, A. C. I., Etim, E. E. 2010. "Extraction and characterization of shear butter oil. *World J. App. Sci. Tech* 2:282-288.

Asuquo, J. E., A. C. I. Anusiem, E. E. Etim. 2012. "Extraction and Characterization of Rubber Seed Oil." *International Journal of Modern Chemistry* 1(3):109-115.

Atabani, A. E., Silitonga, A. S., Ong, H. C., Mahlia, T. M. I., Masjuki, H. H., Badruddin, I. A., Fayaz, H. 2013. "Non–edible vegetable oils: A critical evaluation of oil extraction, fatty acid compositions, biodiesel production, characteristics, engine performance and emissions production." *Renewable Sustainable Energy Rev* 18:211–245.

Basbes S., Blecker C., Deroanne C., Drira N. E., Hamadi A. 2004. "Date seeds: chemical composition and characteristic profiles of the lipid fraction." *Food Chem* 84:577–584.

Bashar Mudhaffar Abdullah., Jumat Salimon. 2009. "Physicochemical Characteristics of Malaysian Rubber (Hevea Brasiliensis) Seed Oil." *European Journal of Scientific Research ISSN 1450-216X* 31(3):437-445.

Camila Martins Garcia, Sergio Teixeira, Leticia Ledo Marciniuk, Ulf Schuchardt. 2008. "Transesterification of soybean oil catalyzed by sulfated zirconia." *Bioresource Technology* 99:6608–6613.

Carraretto C., Macor A., Mirandola A., Stoppato A., Tonon S. 2004. "Biodiesel as alternative fuel: experimental analysis and energetic evaluations." *Energy* 29: 2195–2211.

Dat N. V. et al. 2012. "Biodiesel synthesis from rubber seed oil." *Vietnam Journal of Science* 21(A):105-113.

Eka, H. D., Tajul Aris, Y., Wan Nadiah, W. A. 2010. "Potential use of Malaysian rubber (Hevea brasiliensis) seed as food, feed and biofuel." *International Food Research Journal* 17:527-534.

Gabien M. Babatunde and Wilson G. Pond. 1990. "Nutritive value of Nigerian rubber seed (Hevea Brasiliensis) meal and oil." IV. *Effects of graded levels of rubber seed meal and oil on energy and nitrogen utinization by growing rats.* Elsevier Science Publishers B.V. Amsterdam 7:6-15.

Gandhi V., Cherian K., Mulky M. 1990. "Nutritional and toxicological evaluation of rubber seed oil." *J Am Oil Chem Soc* 67(11):883-886.

Geo E. V., Nagarajan G., Nagalingam B. 2008. "Experiments on behaviour of preheated rubber seed oil in a direct injection diesel engine." *J Energy Inst* 81(3):177-180.

Geo V. E., Nagarajan G., Nagalingam B. 2009. "Experimental investigations to improve the performance of rubber seed oilefueled diesel engine by dual fueling with hydrogen." *Int J Green Energy* 6(4):343-358.

Geo V. E., Nagarajan G., Nagalingam B. 2010. "Studies on improving the performance of rubber seed oil fuel for diesel engine with DEE port injection." *Fuel* 89(11):3559-3567.

Ghana Statistical Service (2011) *Digest of Macroeconomic Data: Statistic abstract 2010*, Accra, Ghana.

Ghandhi V. M., Cherian K. M., Mulky M. J. 1990. "Nutritional and toxicological evaluation of rubber seed oil." *Journal of the American Oil Chemists' Society* 67:883–886.

Gunstone F. D., Harwood J. L., Padley F. B. 1994. *"The lipid hand book. second edition."* Chapman & Hall chemical Database.

Haswin Kaur Gurdeep Singh, Suzana Yusup, Bawadi Abdullah, Kin Wai Cheah, Fathin Nabilah Azmee, Hon Loong Lam. 2017. "Refining of crude rubber seed oil as a feedstock for biofuel production." *Journal of Environmental Management* 203(3):1011-1016.

Hong K. D. Nguyen, Don N. Ta, Ha T. Nguyen. 2016. "Preparation of Cellulose Based Catalyst for Converting Rubber Seed Oil to Biodiesel." *Journal of Applicable Chemistry* 5(4):727-737.

Huei Ruey Ong, Ridzuan Ramli, Md. Maksudur Rahman Khan, Rosli Mohd Yunus. 2016. "The influence of CuO nanoparticle on non-edible rubber seed oil-based alkyd resin preparation and its antimicrobial activity." *Progress in Organic Coatings* 101:245–252.

Ikwuagwu O. E., Ononogbu I. C., Njoku O. U., 2000. "Production of biodiesel using rubber [He6ea brasiliensis (Kunth. Muell.)] seed oil." *Industrial Crops and Products* 12:57–62.

Ikwuagwu O., Ononogbu I., Njoku O. 2000. "Production of biodiesel using rubber [Hevea brasiliensis (Kunth. Muell.)] seed oil." *Industrial Crops* Prod 12(1):57-62.

Iyayi A. F., P. O. Akpaka and U. Ukpeoyibo. 2008. "Rubber seed processing for value-added latex production in Nigeria." ISSN 1991-637X © 2008 *Academic Journals* 17:4-8.

Jamieson G., Baughman W. 1930. "Para rubber seed oil." *J Am Oil Chem Soc* 7(11):419-421.

Jianbai C. 2000. "Rubber seed oil and u-3 fatty acid." *Tropical Agric Sci Technol* 23(1):10-12.

Jianbai C., Meiying H., Xuhua B. 2004. "Study progress on seed oil of rubber Hevea in Yunnan." *Tropical Agric Sci Technol* 27(4):21-24.

Joon Ching Juan, Mohd Ambar Yarmo, Jingchang Zhang. 2009. "Characterization of zirconium sulfate supported on mesoporous molecular sieve HMS catalyst using XRD, XRF and XPS techniques." *Journal of Nuclear and related Technologies* 6(1):297-305.

Junaid Ahmad a, Suzana Yusup, Awais Bokhari, Ruzaimah Nik Mohammad Kamil. 2014. "Study of fuel properties of rubber seed oil-based biodiesel." *Energy Conversion and Management* 78:266–275.

Kaia Roman. 2003. *"From the Fryer to the Fuel Tank – The Complete guide to using vegetable oil as an Alternative fuel."* Joshua Tickell Publications.

Kamalakar K., Amit Kumar Rajak, R. B. N. Prasad, M. S. L. Karuna. 2013. "Rubber seed oil-based biolubricant base stocks: A potential source for hydraulic oils." *Industrial Crops and Products* 51:249–257.

Khan M. A., Yusup S., Ahmad M. M. 2010. "Acid esterification of a high free fatty acid crude palm oil and crude rubber seed oil blend: optimization and parametric analysis." *Biomass Bioenergy* 34(12):1751-1756.

Kovo, A. G., Bawa, A. A. 2007. "Extraction and characterization of oil from Accia niloticia seeds by different solvents." *J. Eng. App. J* 2:572-575.

Kumar, A., Sharma, S. 2011. "Potential non-edible oil resources as biodiesel feedstock: an Indian perspective." *Renewable Sustainable Energy Rev* 15:1791–1800.

Kyari, M. Z. "Extraction and characterization of seed oils." *Int. Agrophysics* 22:139-142.

Mahbub Morshed, Kaniz Ferdous, Maksudur R. Khan, M. S. I. Mazumder, M. A. Islam, Md. T. Uddin. 2011. "Rubber seed oil as a potential source for biodiesel production in Bangladesh." *Fuel* 90:2981–2986.

Masakazu Toda, Atsushi Takagaki, Mai Okamura, Junko N. Kondo, Shigenobu Hayashi, Kazunari Domen, Michikazu Hara. 2005. "Green Chemistry: Biodiesel made with sugar catalyst" *Nature* 438.

Melvin Jose D., Edwin Raj R., Durga Prasad B., Robert Kennedy Z., Mohammed Ibrahim A. 2011. "A multi-variant approach to optimize process parameters for biodiesel extraction from rubber seed oil." *Appl Energy* 88(6):2056-2063.

Morshed M., Ferdous K., Khan M. R., Mazumder M., Islam M., Uddin M. T. 2011. "Rubber seed oil as a potential source for biodiesel production in Bangladesh." *Fuel* 90(10):2981-2986.

O'Brien R. D. 2004. *"Formulating and processing for applications. Second ed."* Washington, DC: CRC press.

Ohikhena et al. 2006. "Small scale industrial application of rubber seed oil in soap manufacture." *Ife Journal of Science* 8(2):207-210.

Okuhara T. 2002. "Water-tolerant solid acid catalysts", *Chem. Rev* 102:3641–3666.

Osagie O. F, Fekarurhobo G. K. 2014. "Cleaning Agent from Natural Rubber Seed Oil (RSO) and Cassava Peels Ash Extract." *Chemistry and Materials Research ISSN 2224- 3224 (Print) ISSN 2225 0956 (Online)* 6(9).

Qianwen C. 1999. "Preliminary research on the chemical compositions of Hevea brasiliensis and its comprehensive utilizations." *J Central South For Univ* 19(4):58-60.

Ramadhas A. S., Jayaraj S., Muraleedharan C. 2005. "Biodiesel production from high FFA rubber seed oil." *Fuel* 84(4):335-340.

Ramadhas A. S., Jayaraj S., Muraleedharan C. 2005. "Biodiesel production from high FFA rubber seed oil" *Fuel* 84:335–340.

Ramadhas A., Jayaraj S., Muraleedharan C. 2005. "Characterization and effect of using rubber seed oil as fuel in the compression ignition engines." *Renew Energy* 30(5):795-803.

Ramadhas A., Jayaraj S., Muraleedharan C. 2008. "Dual fuel mode operation in diesel engines using renewable fuels: rubber seed oil and coir-pith producer gas." *Renew Energy* 33(9):2077-2083.

Ramadhas A., Muraleedharan C., Jayaraj S. 2005. "Performance and emission evaluation of a diesel engine fueled with methyl esters of rubber seed oil." *Renew Energy* 30(12):1789-1800.

Samuel E. Onoji, Sunny E. Iyuke, Anselm I. Igbafe, Diakanua B. Nkazi. 2016. "Rubber seed oil: A potential renewable source of biodiesel for sustainable development in sub-Saharan Africa." *Energy Conversion and Management* 110:125–134.

Satyanarayana M., Muraleedharan C. 2010. "Methyl ester production from rubber seed oil using two-step pretreatment process." *Int J Green Energy* 7(1):84-90.

Satyanarayana M., Muraleedharan C. 2011. "A comparative study of vegetable oil methyl esters (biodiesels)." *Energy* 36(4):2129-2137.

Satyanarayana M., Muraleedharan C. 2011. "Comparative studies of biodiesel production from rubber seed oil, coconut oil, and palm oil including thermogravimetric analysis." *Energy Sour Part Recovery Util Environ Eff* 33(10):925-937.

Shuli Yan, Craig DiMaggio, Siddharth Mohan, Manhoe Kim, Steven O. Salley, K. Y. Simon Ng. 2010. "Advancements in Heterogeneous Catalysis for Biodiesel Synthesis." *Top Catal* 53:721–736.

Smith K., El-Hiti G. A., Jayne A. J., Butters M. 2003. "Acetylation of aromatic ethers using acetic anhydride over solid acid catalysts in a solvent-free system. Scope of the reaction for substituted ethers." *Org. Biomol. Chem* 1:1560–1564.

Toda, M., Takagaki, A., Okamura, M., Kondo, J. N., Hayashi, S., Domen, K., and Hara, M. 2005. "Green chemistry - Biodiesel made with sugar catalyst." *Nature* 438(7065):178.

Victor Shang-Yi Lin et al. 2010. "Porous Silica and metal oxide composite-based catalyst for conversion of fatty acids and oils to biodiesel." *US* 7790651 B2.

Weiwei L., Youyong S., Wudi Z., Shiqing L., Chaofeng X. 2005. "Preparation of biodiesel fuel with rubber seed oil." *China Oils Fats* 30(10):63-66.

Wendy Pei Qin Ng, Hon Loong Lam, Suzana Yusup. 2013. "Supply network synthesis on rubber seed oil utilisation as potential biofuel feedstock." *Energy* 55:82-88.

Wu C., Yin X., Yuan Z., Zhou Z., Zhuang X. 2010. "The development of bioenergy technology in China." *Energy* 35(11):4445-4450.

Wuttichai Roschat, Theeranun Siritanon, Boonyawan Yoosuk, Taweesak Sudyoadsuk, Vinich Promarak. 2017. "Rubber seed oil as potential non-edible feedstock for biodiesel production using heterogeneous catalyst in Thailand." *Renewable Energy* 101:937-944.

Xiankun L., Changjiu S., Bohuang L. 2009. "Development and utilization of biodiesel extracted from rubber seed." *Tropical Agric Sci Technol* 32(2):14-16.

Yang R, Su M., Zhang J., Jin F., Zha C., Li M., et al. 2011. "Biodiesel production from rubber seed oil using poly (sodium acrylate) supporting NaOH as a water-resistant catalyst." *Bioresour Technol* 102(3):2665-2671.

Yixin Zhu, Jianchu Xu, Qiaohong Li, Peter E. Mortimer. 2014. "Investigation of rubber seed yield in Xishuangbanna and estimation of rubber seed oil-based biodiesel potential in Southeast Asia." *Energy* 69(1):837-842.

Yong O. Y., Jumat S. 2006. "Characteristics of Elateriospermum tapos seed oil as a new source of oilseed." *Industrial Crops and Products* 24:146-151.

Yong O. Y., Salimon J. 2006. "Characteristics of Elateriospermum tapos seed oil as a new source of oilseed." *Ind Crop Prod* 24:146–151.

Yusup S., Khan M. 2010. "Basic properties of crude rubber seed oil and crude palm oil blend as a potential feedstock for biodiesel production with enhanced cold flow characteristics." *Biomass Bioenergy* 34(10):1523-1526.

Zhao P., An F., Yu X., Peng M. 2008. "Progress on exploitation and utilization of rubber seeds." *Chin J Tropical Agric* 2.

About the Editor

Assoc. Prof. Hong K.D. Nguyen is an Associate Professor in Organic and Petrol Chemical Engineering, School of Chemical Engineering, Ha Noi University of Science and Technology (HUST).

She got her PhD in Chemistry from University College London in 2007 and was promoted as Youngest Associate Professor of Viet Nam in 2012. She was awarded Gold medal of The World Intellectual Property Organization Award for the Best Young Inventor of Viet Nam in 2003, First Prize of Viet Nam Intellectual Forum of Technology (VIFOTEC) for creative scientific research in 2008. She is particularly interested in (1) novel technologies and methodologies, novel material processes, chemical processes for green products from biomass, (2) preparation and characterization of new materials/heterogeneous catalyst especially aspects of composition and structure, (3) Applying and transferring researches into the industry. (4) Green Energy, Bio-fuels, green fuels from vegetable oil and biomass.

Prof Hong has been the PI of over 10 projects funded by the Newton Fund United Kingdom, British Council United Kingdom, Vietnam Ministry of Science and technology, Vietnam Ministry of Industry & Trade, Vietnam Ministry of Transport, Vietnam National Oil and Gas group.

INDEX

A

D

E

F

G

H

I

J

K

L

M

P

T

U

V

W

X

Y

Z

B